Liz—
Thank you for trusting me with
Alexa's care—
Marianne Uebang

MIND
AND
MEDICINE:

IN
HARMONY
FOR
HEALING!

MIND AND MEDICINE:

IN HARMONY FOR HEALING!

DR. MARIANNE MURRAY URBANSKI

LIFESUCCESS PUBLISHING, LLC
8900 E. Pinnacle Peak Road, Suite D240
Scottsdale, AZ 85255

Telephone:	800.473.7134
Fax:	480.661.1014
E-mail:	admin@lifesuccesspublishing.com
ISBN:	978-1-59930-323-9
Cover:	Lloyd Arbour, LifeSuccess Publishing, LLC
Text:	Lloyd Arbour, LifeSuccess Publishing, LLC
Edit:	LifeSuccess Publishing, LLC; Publication Services

COMPANIES, ORGANIZATIONS, INSTITUTIONS, AND INDUSTRY PUBLICATIONS. Quantity discounts are available on bulk purchases of this book for reselling, educational purposes, subscription incentives, gifts, sponsorship, or fundraising. Special books or book excerpts can also be created to fit specific needs such as private labeling with your logo on the cover and a message from a VIP printed inside. For more information, please contact our Special Sales Department at LifeSuccess Publishing, LLC.

Printed in Canada.

Dedication

I want to dedicate this book to three people who have profoundly impacted my life.

To my mother, Edna Murray, who dedicated her life to her children: You taught me more through your illness and death than most people can teach in an entire lifetime.

To my father, William J. Murray Jr., MD, who dedicated his life to his children and his patients: You taught me how to treat my patients with compassion and respect.

To my sister, and best friend, Carolyn Murray, who dedicated her life to serving others. Through her career as a nurse and friend, she touched the lives of so many people in her short life. I truly believe the world is a better place because she was here: You taught me that if I believed in myself, I could accomplish anything.

To these three people, who I will always love and keep close in my heart: I thank you for encouraging me to share my ideas and inspiring me to fulfill my dream.

Foreword

Dr. Marianne Urbanski explores the power of the mind to heal bodies while working in harmony with modern medicine. Anyone who has ever been a patient or supported a friend or family member who was a patient will benefit from the wisdom and insights shared in *Mind & Medicine.*

Due to her unique point of view as a periodontist, Dr. Urbanski helps patients and families understand the powerful connection of the subconscious and conscious minds and how they work together to heal the body. She exposes how limiting beliefs are engrained in our minds as children and how we can move beyond those learned behaviors and ideas to create a new and healthy life.

Every reader will feel the empowerment they have within to understand their own thoughts and learn to use those thoughts to help their bodies. By examining the universal laws and showing how to apply them in everyday life, Dr. Urbanski gives the reader the tools and knowledge to initiate change within themselves and those around them. She shows how so many barriers, including those associated with our health, are self-created and can be overcome once our perspective is altered.

Friends and family members can also learn how their thoughts impact a loved one who is ill or struggling with disease. *Mind & Medicine* reveals that family members and medical professionals have the opportunity to create a positive and healing environment for the patient and can directly impact the healing that the patient experiences.

Don't hesitate to absorb every page of this wonderful book and put it to work instantly in your life. It makes no difference if you are struggling with a terminal illness, if you are experiencing minor health issues, or if you are trying to prevent them; this book can make a world of difference in your life.

—Bob Proctor,
featured in _The Secret_ and author of _You Were Born Rich_

Acknowledgments

There are many people who I would like to thank for their help during this process.

To all of the people at LifeSuccess, thank you for your guidance on this exciting new journey.

To my "Q force" friends, Simon Marples, Joan McAndrews and Kathy Fiedler, thank you for keeping me motivated, challenged and "on track" every week.

To Joan McAndrews, a special thank you for inspiring me and being instrumental in the creation of this book.

To my fantastic staff, Sandy, Jennifer, Brenda, Dorrie, and Sara, thank you for being the best people to work with in the entire world.

To my patients, thank you for allowing me to serve you and for trusting me to provide periodontal care.

To my siblings, Patti, Ellen, Gloria, Edna and Bill, thank you for your unending encouragement and support.

To Bill, thank you for your inspiration, encouragement and most importantly, your love.

To my children, Laura and John, thank you both for bringing joy to my life everyday.

Finally, thank you to all the people that contributed to the book by sharing their stories with me. I couldn't have written this without their input.

Contents

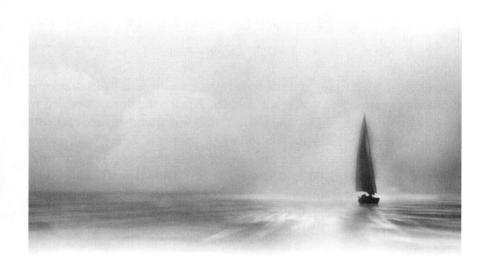

Chapter One

—Your Health at Risk—

*In order to change we must be sick
and tired of being sick and tired.*

—Author Unknown

Chapter One

Rhonda had been ill on and off for several months and had undergone numerous treatments for her gall bladder. Finally, the doctor decided to remove the offending organ, and all her family and friends waited excitedly in the waiting room for the good news. A couple of hours later, a very groggy Rhonda awoke to the teary faces of those she loved. Her husband, Mike, squeezed her hand as new tears flowed. She knew it wasn't good. The doctor entered the room and a quiet hush fell on everyone present. "It's cancer," he said. Rhonda heard only bits and pieces of the conversation that included the words malignant, inoperable, and months.

I visited her several times over the next two weeks and watched helplessly as she became a mere shell of the vivacious and funny person she had once been. The room was always quiet, and her family whispered and cried frequently with her. They talked about funeral arrangements and how the children would be taken care of. The doctors seemed stunned at her rapid decline, but it made sense to me. Rhonda was surrounded by the energy of death every second of every day after the diagnosis was delivered. In essence, she'd already decided that there was no option other than death. Rather than choosing to fight, or even get another opinion, she released all hope and embraced what she saw as her fate. She died exactly two weeks later at the age of 48. There was no medical reason for her rapid decline as the doctors were convinced she could have easily lived for months at the very least. The only thing that changed was her mind-set.

The mind is incredibly powerful and can easily accomplish what doctors and medicine can never duplicate or explain. As far back as the 1880s medical science has known of something called the placebo effect. In essence, it is the ability of the body to heal itself or gain improvement physically once the mind is convinced that a particular treatment or drug is effective. As many physicians are now discovering, the mind has even more impact on our physical well-being than initially assumed. Andrew's experience with a devastating diagnosis highlights how the mind can be our biggest ally.

In the winter of 1983 while chopping wood at our cabin, I felt a sharp pain in my right hand. Over the next few hours my right side then my left side went numb from head to toe, and my coordination was a little off. I was scared I might be experiencing the first signs of a stroke, and I was only 32. I went to my doctor immediately, and he scheduled an emergency MRI. It was right around the holidays, and I remember fear overwhelming me at the idea that this could be my last Christmas. The next evening, the neurologist called my home and asked me and my wife to come to his office first thing Monday morning. He said it wasn't a stroke or a brain tumor, but he also didn't say what it was. That night was the longest night of my life, and I didn't sleep a wink. I had three young daughters and wanted to see them grow up, get married, and have babies of their own.

The next morning, the doctor took over an hour telling us everything that wasn't wrong with me. Finally after he went down the list he told me it was MS. He suggested that I prepare myself for death or to be in a wheelchair within ten years. His whole attitude angered me—was I just supposed to give up and die? I told the doctor that the diagnosis was his opinion and that I wasn't going to wait around for it to happen.

I sat alone for a long time after we returned home. I visualized myself healthy and active at the age of 85. I imagined my girls graduating college and my grandchildren sitting on my lap. I made a list of the things I planned to do like skydiving, rock climbing, and taking my wife on a European vacation. Most of all, I convinced myself that I could beat this disease and live a full and long life.

Needless to say, my doctor was skeptical and not very supportive of what I was doing. I realized his negative attitude was affecting me each and every time I saw him, as he was completely resigned to what he believed was inevitable. So I changed doctors. My symptoms improved, and I continued with life.

About five years later I applied for an insurance policy, and they required another MRI. The new test showed that 90 percent of the previous scar tissue was gone. The new neurologist said that wasn't supposed to happen and I still had MS, but he couldn't explain the improvement. I have never owned the illness, nor do I consciously think of myself as sick in any way.

This coming winter will mark the 25th year since the first diagnosis. In that time I have climbed mountains on three continents, earned a pilot's license, traveled to Europe many times with my wife, and rejoiced at the birth of each of my eight grandchildren. I look back on my diagnosis as one of the greatest gifts I could have been given. It galvanized my positive attitude and made me decide what I really wanted my life to be.

Physical impairment and death can be very difficult for doctors to deal with and hard to discuss with patients. Physicians can react to the impending death of their patients with powerful emotions, and patients can't help but be affected by these emotions. Physicians often fear losing control and realize that at some point they will not be able to help their patient any further. This inadequacy of human ability can produce feelings of helplessness in people. The reason many students enter medical school is to gain the ability and knowledge to make a difference where others cannot. When this reality reaches its limit, many physicians find themselves in an unfamiliar, very uncomfortable situation that can project very negative emotions toward the patient.

Doctors are people too. They have their own experiences, their own fears, and their own lack of belief to conquer. They do not know everything, nor can they accurately predict what will or won't happen. They can give us odds and percentages, but they can't say for certain where we will fall in that range or if those odds will even apply. But we still place a great deal of emphasis on what they say in regard to our health and even our death.

Our attitude affects every part of our lives, not only our health, but our results in *all* aspects of our lives: relationships, personal growth, financial success, and so many more areas. Have you ever noticed that some people succeed at almost everything they try, while others seem to have a dark cloud shadowing their efforts at every turn? Similarly, how many times have you been shocked by someone you assumed to be an active middle-aged person only to learn that they are in their 70 or even 80s?

The people who succeed in business and other areas of life know how to program their minds for success, while others may be operating under negative suggestions or beliefs developed early in life that inhibit their outcomes. Everything we are, or do, is a result of what we think and believe. Numerous studies of children have shown that those who were told they were smart believed this to be true, and their grades were excellent. Those that were reprimanded and told they were not able to get good grades believed that as well, and sadly, it affected their lives negatively for years to come.

As we grow we learn certain limitations about what is possible for us from what we were told and from our own life experiences. Something can be so far outside of our experience that it would not even occur to us to think of it. It would seem to be an impossible fantasy.

Although we may think that our health is separate from these concerns, it is actually very much affected by what we think and feel. Dangerous and even life-threatening conditions such as high blood pressure, digestive problems, and heart disease are brought on or aggravated by stress—and stress is a perception of the mind. We have the ability to decide if and when we feel stressed, and how we deal with that stress affects our long term health.

It is also true that positive emotions increase longevity and lower these risk factors. This is why people in long-term relationships have overall better health than those who are not. It also points to why activities such as pet therapy in hospitals and nursing homes have been so effective. People perceive their lives to be better through the interaction with others and even with pets, and therefore they live happier, healthier lives.

One of the newer fields of research is psychoneuroimmunology, which is the study of the connection between behavior, neural, and endocrine function and immune processes. A colleague of mind, David Yeo, is a professor and head athletic trainer at Eastern Connecticut State University. He has written articles on the mind/body connection and states, "Because the mind and body are inextricably linked, attitudes, beliefs, and emotions can trigger chain reactions that affect blood chemistry and the activity of every cell and organ system."

This has tremendous implications for those who are consistently in a negative or unhealthy state of mind. Yeo also states, "In the brain, positive beliefs and expectations produce biochemical and physiological changes. Positive emotions can produce neuropeptides that protect the tissues and act to ward off disease and facilitate recovery." Doctors have long set aside the patient's emotional state and have focused on the physical state. This research conveys the idea that not only does the mind have the ability to heal; it also has the ability to protect the body from disease.

The idea that animals make many of us feel good is also supported by physiological data. Studies examining heart rate and stress chemicals, for example, showed that even relatively brief interactions with a pet (usually dogs) produced measurable beneficial effects. Longer-term interactions, such as pet ownership or companionship, have been found to result in positive cardiac outcomes, such as living longer and recovering faster after a heart attack than non-owners. Elderly animal owners were also found to make fewer visits to their doctors, even during times of stress.

People with good emotional health are aware of their thoughts, feelings, and behaviors. They have learned healthy ways to cope with the stress and the problems that are a normal part of life. They feel good about themselves and have healthy relationships. However, many things that happen in our lives can disrupt this balance of emotional health and lead to strong feelings of sadness, stress, or anxiety. These things could include:

Serious illness

Empty nest—or return to the nest

Loss of a loved one

Divorce or marriage

Job change or promotions

Financial problems

Birth of a child

Buying a new home

It is important to note that often positive changes, such as the birth of a child, can be just as stressful as negative changes. During these times of great change in our lives, the body responds to the way we think, feel, and act. This is often referred to as the "mind/body connection." When we are stressed, anxious, or upset, our body experiences changes such as the release of certain hormones and enzymes that are the body's signals that something isn't right. For example, high blood pressure or a stomach ulcer might develop after a particularly stressful event, such as the death of a loved one.

Unfortunately, many people live in what they perceive to be an ongoing state of stress. This poor emotional health can weaken our body's immune system, making us more likely to get colds and other infections during emotionally difficult times. Also, when we are feeling stressed, anxious, or upset, we may not take care of our health as well as we should. We may not feel like exercising, eating nutritious foods, or taking medicine that the doctor prescribes. Abuse of alcohol, tobacco, or other drugs may also be a sign of poor emotional health.

I've stated that stress is largely a problem of perception. We can think of perception like wearing a particular set of glasses through which we view every experience in our lives. These perceptions are created from the ideas we were raised with. These ideas may have come from teachers, parents, and any authority figure that we associated with in our youth. They are also formed by events that happen in our lives. These events are more traumatic when we are young, but events can also affect us as adults, and these events shape our perception from that point forward.

This change in perspective can be either positive or negative. If we are presented with a crisis, as Andrew was, we can choose to believe what is presented, or we can choose to reject their idea of reality and create our own. To Rhonda, however, this didn't even seem possible. She accepted her fate without question. The idea that there might be a choice didn't even enter her thought process. Why?

Throughout this book, we will examine the components of how our perceptions are created and how we can change them. We may feel that we don't have control of our thoughts and can't understand how we would change. But the ideas we may have had for decades aren't as set in stone as we might think, and I will show that they are merely our perception. We each have the ability to change our lives, no matter what our age is or what our life experiences are. Through the years, the medical community has relegated the idea that the mind is powerful enough to heal to the fringes of accepted medicine. Only in the past decade has western medicine been more accepting of the idea that the brain, and more specifically our thoughts, can have a positive effect on our overall health. While negative emotions such as those we associate with anxiety and depression (often generally contributed to stress) have long been identified as the culprit in many chronic patterns of disease, the idea that positive emotions could have a healing effect has been pushed aside until recently.

Now as more research is being conducted in the field known as psychoneuroimmunology—the of the interaction of the mind and the effect thoughts can have on the immune system—it is even more clear that the attitude and beliefs held by a person can affect their health and longevity.

We become what we think about. This fact has been accepted for literally centuries, dating back and even preceding the Greek philosophers. The power of the mind has always been a source of fascination, but in our world of great medical advances and technological breakthroughs, the power of the mind has been discounted and set aside.

We have been conditioned to allow our thoughts to run rampant, often leading to less than stellar results. Our thoughts are very critical with respect to achieving our goals and dreams, so it is important to understand the processes that govern our thinking. The beliefs we currently have don't just happen. They are cumulative over time, and they change frequently.

Though we have the capacity to understand highly complex and abstract ideas, when we think it is often as though a movie scenario runs through our minds. When we are young we learn to communicate by associating words with pictures. We see everything in fabulous Technicolor rather than snowy black and white. The pictures we make in our mind start with a single thought, which is expounded upon and then finalized as a physical entity. Words, in and of themselves, are vague and have only the meaning we give them through these pictures. When I say the word RED, we see the color red in our mind's eye. The reason we associate the word and color together is through learning and conditioning. We could call the color red PURPLE and it would still be just as red. We learned to associate the word red and that particular color together. We freely associate ideas and circumstances all the time.

When we strive to achieve something, it makes a difference whether or not we have a clear mental picture of the outcome we want. Our mental clarity helps create the life, health, and wealth that we want to enjoy. The clearer the picture, the more effective it is. I've learned through my own experiences and working with patients that when our thoughts are focused, we experience a more fulfilled life with less fear, doubt, and confusion. But when negative thoughts or panic sets in during a crisis it becomes a downward spiral of fear and doubt.

This entire process occurs in our minds and is our perception of the situation. What do you think of when I ask you to "think of your mind?" Most of us will probably imagine a picture of the brain. But our brain is not our mind. Our mind is actually an activity of cells that are found in all of our being, and since no one has actually seen the mind, we are going to create a picture of the mind to work with. This picture is the stick person and was first introduced by Dr. Thurman Fleet in the 1930s. He was very involved in the healing arts, and he said: "You know, if we're just treating the body, we're treating symptoms. If we're going to treat the cause of the problems, we've got to go beyond that." He used this picture to help us understand how we need to look at the behavior and thoughts to change our results. Now, don't let the simplicity of this drawing fool you. I think this picture is so profound, and I have learned so much studying it, I would like to share it with you.

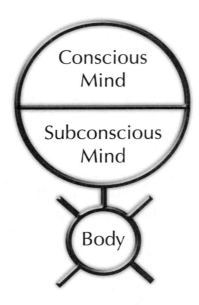

As we can see in this illustration, the mind is disproportionately larger than the body. This is because the mind creates what we experience through our bodies. We can divide the mind into two parts: the conscious or thinking mind, and the subconscious mind, or the feeling mind. The thinking mind is where our thoughts originate. We have the ability to accept, reject, or neglect our thoughts. The conscious mind allows us to choose which thoughts we agree with and which we don't. The accepted thoughts take up residence in our subconscious as new ideas or as confirmation of existing beliefs.

For example, if someone told us that the earth is flat, we would reject the idea because it doesn't agree with what we already know to be true. In our conscious mind not only do we have the power to choose our thoughts, but we also have the ability to focus on the positive or negative side of a situation. It is the conscious mind that can look at a situation objectively and decide how we respond to new circumstances, and this can be hard, especially when faced with the unknown. Many times, because our subconscious mind is our feeling mind, we respond with emotion at first. For example, if a loved one is diagnosed with cancer we usually would naturally respond emotionally to the news and then later think about how we will handle the situation. As we increase awareness of how our own limiting beliefs play into those decisions, we are able to consciously choose a positive response. We will discuss how this is done in subsequent chapters.

The bottom part of the diagram shows the subconscious mind. This emotional portion of the mind is the culmination of the ideas that the conscious mind has accepted over time as reality. The subconscious mind is where we hold our beliefs, habits, and our self image. If at one point our conscious mind accepted the idea that we weren't intelligent, then when the subconscious is confronted with the statement, "You are a genius," we immediately reject it because it doesn't agree with what the subconscious mind is telling us.

While the earth being round is a simple example, think of the ramifications for other ideas that we have accepted as reality; ideas such as "I'm not the healthy type," or "I'm not supposed to feel good at this age," or even "I am old" (a negative association with that). These negative ideas, sometimes called limiting beliefs, can also be firmly established in the subconscious and can cause us to reject statements and ideas that could help us live healthier, happier lives.

It is important to understand that the subconscious mind cannot differentiate between real and imagined. One of the most effective tools for patients recovering from or coping with disease or chronic illness is visualization. They visualize themselves feeling wonderful and being able to live normal lives again. As they intensely visualize these scenes of recovery in their minds, the subconscious mind accepts them as though they are happening right now. This has tremendous healing power because remember, what we think about, we become. If we think about death and dying, it comes to us. If we think about good health and living, it comes to us as well. That which we think about, we will become.

While the stick person appears to be a simple and easy illustration, it is actually very powerful and can enlighten us toward possibility. The most critical step in understanding the power of our thoughts is to become aware of them. As we are bombarded with literally thousands of thoughts per day, we choose which ones we accept. This new awareness brings to light any self-limiting thoughts that are emanating from our subconscious that we may want to change.

Our choice of thought directly affects our feelings, which then affects our actions and the results we experience. Therefore, if we want to change our results, we must start with our conscious thoughts. If we actively choose positive thoughts, then we will invoke positive feelings. The Law of Polarity states that is literally impossible to have positive thoughts and at the same time have negative feelings and vice versa. If our thoughts focus on the negative things that happen during the course of each day we will not only feel terrible, we will attract more of the same. This isn't just about our state of mind; it is also about our state of health, and I feel the most effective way to improve our health is to start with our mind.

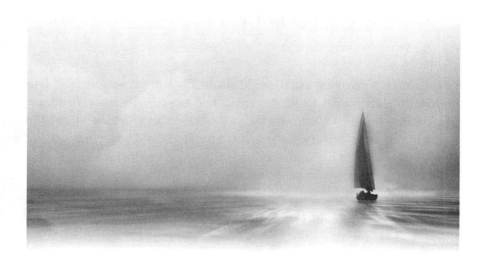

Chapter Two

—You Already Have Belief Systems—

Belief is the basis of all action, and,
this being so, the belief that dominates the
hearts or mind is shown in the life.

—from *Above Life's Turmoil*

Chapter Two

Leslie became a widow after her husband died unexpectedly. She had nothing in place, and their life insurance had lapsed. The apartment lease was coming to an end, and she did not have enough money to pay the next month's rent. Leslie sank into a deep depression, believing that she was helpless without her husband, and moreover, hopeless at being able to succeed in raising her three children alone.

Due to this attitude, she was ill much of the time, worrying over every small detail as she doubted her ability to be an effective single mother. The thought of raising three children between ages ten and sixteen weighed heavily on her, and it showed in her physical appearance as she actually became fragile and her body appeared like a woman ten or even twenty years older. The self-image she once held of herself, a confident, strong-willed woman, grew dim. Every move she made seemed like the wrong one to her. She questioned everything she thought she knew.

Leslie's self-image was that of a wife and mother, and now that her husband was gone and her skills as a mother were fading as well, her present confidence and beliefs were faltering.

Unfortunately, this is an all too common scenario, and it reiterates that our belief systems, how we are raised, what we are told, and who we believe ourselves to be are perceptions that can be changed—and in Leslie's case, shaken to the core. Her thoughts—nothing else—had affected her mental state and her overall health and appearance. She was on a downward spiral, the same spiral that many people experience who are grieving or dealing with long-term illness or chronic disease.

Our belief systems are very strong and are an accumulation of things we've been told, read, or learned throughout our lives. In order to understand the complexity of beliefs, let's take a look at a developing mind—a baby's mind. We know how vulnerable their little minds can be. They are like sponges, absorbing and repeating every word and action they see. It is amazing when we think of the influence that parents and even other authority figures, like teachers, have on children.

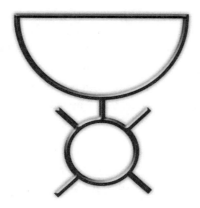

At birth our mind is wide open, and thoughts, images, and ideas go directly into the subconscious mind without being filtered by the conscious mind. These beliefs become fixed in our subconscious minds as truth. We have no real reasoning ability or filter at this stage, so we accept everything as reality. The subconscious mind cannot distinguish between real and imagined, so without the filter of the conscious mind, these beliefs become automatically accepted as true, and they are carried with us into our adult years.

All through childhood our mind is being conditioned, and our self-image is being formed. This includes accepting whatever label is given to us or we give to ourselves. These could include labels such as smart, pretty, stupid, ugly, and many others. We retain those labels and ideas as truth even though they may stem from one comment or one small incident on the playground.

It is during this very critical time in the development of the child when our paradigms and belief systems are formed. Paradigms can be defined as a philosophical or theoretical framework or a pattern of behavior, thought, or actions. We tend to have the same paradigms as those people who are the most influential in our lives.

Events throughout life can change and alter our perception of ourselves, and we can choose to accept or reject new ideas. This is especially true when hardship, death, illness, or anything outside the realm of everyday routine comes to the foreground. The possibility for the mind to develop and change existing ideas is present—but we choose whether those changes will be positive or negative. The mind never stops, so the possibility for progression never stops.

The mind is more absorbent in the early stages of life before we develop our conscious mind, which is really our ability to reason. Think about the way an infant smiles or the way they stare. They are taking us in. They are taking the world in. They are absorbing everything they can and depositing that into their subconscious mind. As the child grows they see how their father behaves with their mother, if he is gentle when he interacts with her or if he yells when something is done unfavorably—this same behavior will most likely turn up again later in life of that child either through their own actions or their choice of relationships. We tend to repeat and relive what we see as a child.

It is important to understand that belief systems do not develop strictly from negative experiences. Positive experiences also help develop our belief system as well. We can have great success in grade school or in sports at a young age which may convince us that we can accomplish anything. Or we can witness a wonderful giving relationship between our parents, which encourages us to seek out a similar situation for ourselves.

Unfortunately, many people tend to dwell on the mishaps or the negativity of life rather than focusing on the good. In general, we relay negative news far more frequently than positive, we worry about bad situations happening far more than we look forward to good, and it is critical to remember that the thoughts we choose are our choice. We look back on New Year's Eve and we make resolutions to improve what we failed on last year. We say we will eat better, we will exercise more, we will take better care of our health. Rarely do I ever hear someone say, "I'm going to keep reading to my children," or, "I'm going to keep biking to work instead of driving." We create habits of verbalizing and dwelling on negativity in our lives, and this affects everything we do and everything we feel. We remember negativity more readily due to this repetition, and we forget how these positive influences affect and mold our belief system. However, occasionally a positive incident influences our future, and this is wonderful!

For example, a friend of mine named Dane told me a story of an incident when he was twelve years old. He was walking behind his grandmother and grandfather. His brother was walking beside him. They came from a good home, but were never intentionally instructed how to act proper, sincere, or genuine. Instead, these were taught by example. On this particular day, he said, the town was quiet. The sun's rays followed the length of the street, throwing long shadows across the pavement. He remembers watching his grandfather and thinking how he strode with pride—the way he held himself. He also recalled the way he looked ahead and never at the ground with his long gait, and how he and his brother had to take five steps for their grandfather's one.

My friend remembers his grandmother's hand and how it was placed neatly in the fold of his grandfather's elbow. She wore a blue dress, and her hair was done just so. She had a calm look on her face when she turned around and said, "Do you see how your grandpa always walks on the street side of the sidewalk?" Dane said he remembers his brother nodding and how his grandfather turned his head to him slightly and winked, as if it were a secret.

Years later, after both boys grew up and had children of their own, they were picnicking together in the country and his brother said, "Do you remember that day when Grandma and Grandpa took us out and she told me that Grandpa always walks on the street side?" His brother laughed and said, "I still can't walk on the inside of the sidewalk with my wife. It just seems wrong."

This appears to be such a small incident and seemingly meaningless to outsiders, but that one small comment from my friend's grandmother completely changed the way they both walk down the street with their wives to this day. To the developing mind, no incident, good or bad, would be seen as insignificant. The baby's mind accepts everything as true. This is the way our subconscious mind is strongly influenced by our parents and grandparents. This is how many of our habits and paradigms are formed.

I love hearing stories like that, stories where so much can be learned, retained, developed, and then used and reused repeatedly throughout one's life. It was a moment in Dane's life that affected his mental health and attitude in a positive manner. Dane now has two boys of his own and will no doubt share that tradition with them.

All through our lives we are influenced by many factors. People we meet, places we go, the money we make, the things we succeed at, the challenges we may or may not have met—all of these have their effects on the way we live our lives and whether we allow these things to have a positive influence on us. It is not solely our opinions that define who we are, but the actions that result from these ingrained beliefs, and for better or worse, these actions create our results.

Leslie, who lost her husband, was not a weak-willed woman. She knew how to be a good parent. But losing her husband, trying to raise three children, and working two jobs left her feeling inadequate when she was anything but this. In her mind she carried her many ideals, dreams, hopes, and ambitions: she wanted her children to go to good schools, and she wanted to travel with her late husband, live on a lake, and drink her coffee on the deck in the morning with him and watch the sun come up while the water was still silent. This is what her subconscious mind wanted and what she dreamed of.

But the shock of his death shattered her confidence, and she was overtaken by doubt and fear. Her paradigm was challenged, and soon her inaction and maternal doubts manifested. These thoughts were ingrained in her subconscious mind, and this became her new self-image. She was no longer a woman enjoying peaceful mornings overlooking the lake, but instead she was a woman questioning her ability to raise her children.

I ran into her a few months after her husband had died. She looked ragged. The loss had taken its toll on her appearance. Deep and dark circles ran under eyes, and I could tell the crying had not yet waned. The constant questioning and doubting had taken a severe toll on her mental health. And then, almost without warning, Leslie looked at me and asked, "Why did this happen?" Right there on the sidewalk Leslie told me what she had wanted to become and what she wanted for her children. The Leslie I remembered had wanted only to grow old with this man that she loved so dearly. But now her inactions and incessant hesitation seemed to be controlled by everyone but her. Leslie mistakenly thought that the circumstances had produced these problems, but in truth her own thoughts had.

Problems and circumstances will always arise, and challenges must always be met. One reason it is difficult to pull back into a positive state is that the deeper one slides, the greater the struggle seems to climb back up, but we do have that choice. We do have the option to take control of our actions. We have the choice to decide who we are and who we will become. I shared this idea with Leslie, and naturally she took it with skepticism because her self-image had fallen so far. Taking control of our thoughts involves becoming responsible for our thoughts and actions and tapping into our higher thought faculties. I realize it appears like I am implying that this is an easy process. It is absolutely not, but it is one that is possible for us all, and it is this process of learning how to alter our thoughts and choose the thoughts we allow to enter into our conscious minds that we will discuss throughout this book. This decline of self image happens almost without notice and not only if we experience a negative situation, such as death of a loved one or if we learn that we have a new chronic illness. Our subconscious minds are also impacted by the things we watch on television and the people we spend our time with. There is a very tenuous time when the decision to focus on the positive side of the situation or slide into the pit of negativity is critical.

By letting these negative thoughts enter the subconscious mind, we can become angry and hateful. It is then easy to place the blame on people and things that are completely innocent or who have no control over the situation. We have the ability to choose whether or not to allow circumstances to control our emotions in a very negative way. These negative emotions are then picked up and transferred to those around us. This occurs through our vibration. Each emotion we produce sends out a vibration. This is picked up by others and we literally attract those with a like mind-set.

Our outward demeanor gives signals and clues to those around us. Therefore, our results are not a reflection of our potential; they are a result of the thoughts we allow into the conscious mind. This is a critical point. By choosing positive thoughts, our feelings toward a given situation will reflect a positive outlook and this is marked by fewer and less severe emotional outbursts. Heightened negative emotions are a good sign that our thoughts are not on a positive path. If we get overly angry or upset in a certain situation, that is a hint to look more closely at what is going on with our thoughts.

The Law of Polarity tells us that it is impossible to have negative feelings and positive thoughts at the same time. If we consciously focus on the positive, we will be able to favorably affect those around us. This is why it is so important for patients, physicians and family members to express hope and optimism. Family members and the medical community work together, and if one person demonstrates a negative or uncertain outlook, this can be extremely detrimental to the outcome of the patient.

Our body is the instrument of the mind. The information and decisions that come from our conscious and subconscious mind move the body to take action. Accordingly, the actions we take and the behavior we engage in will ultimately give us the results we see in our lives, but this all starts with our thoughts.

An example of how our thoughts can negatively affect our health is if we allow primarily pessimistic thoughts into our conscious mind, then these will pass through the subconscious mind and will have a negative effect on our body. This can manifest through our health as high blood pressure, ulcers, tension headaches, and a number of other conditions .

The link between a person's overall attitude and their health is very strong. By focusing and visualizing what we want instead of accepting limiting beliefs we have learned throughout our lives, we can make a substantial and sustainable change in our lives.

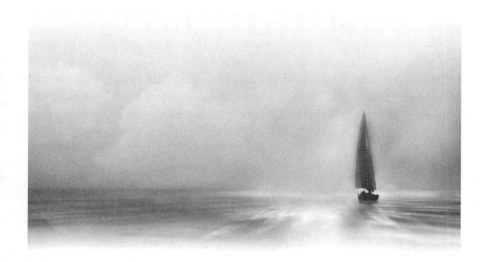

Chapter Three

—Mind Is What Matters—

Whatever the mind can conceive,
it can achieve.

—from *The Secret*

Chapter Three

Once we gain an awareness that our conscious mind is the filter, we can then learn to evaluate thoughts before they can affect us. We can literally choose to accept or reject thoughts in this dimension. In order to do this, we must understand how these thoughts enter the conscious mind.

The Five Senses

The primary way most people receive information about their world is through the use of their five senses. These senses take in our world and transmit that data to our conscious mind. They are "hard wired" to our minds and function almost like small antennae.

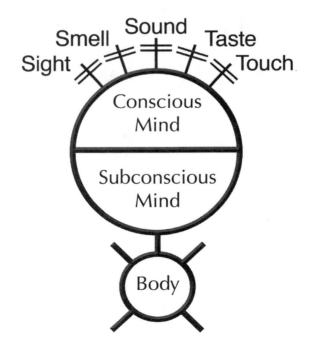

The five senses are: sight, smell, taste, hearing, and touch. They constantly work to bring information about our world into our minds. That information affects how and what we think. For example, we hear a bit of bad news and we instantly become sad. Similarly, we might smell a certain type of perfume and remember a certain person or experience we had in our past. Our emotions are constantly changing in response to the information from the five senses. But we can choose how this occurs by choosing the thoughts we allow the conscious mind to accept. If a negative thought enters our mind, we can reject the idea and refocus on something positive. However, this takes practice, especially if we've been habitually unconditionally accepting information from the senses for a long while.

The subconscious mind is the storage facility for information accepted by our conscious mind and also for all the information gained from our life experiences, what we've been taught, and what we've read.

There is a natural priority for how the information is sorted within the human mind. Things that can be physically threatening are priority and are hard wired into our mind so that if we are faced with a threat, any critical information needed in an instant is available to us. For example, if we can't swim and suddenly find ourselves in deep water, our instinct takes over and we attempt to at least dog paddle for survival. The information we need to know is made available immediately to activate our flight or fight response and save us from harm. The problem here is that our fear usually causes us to act irrationally, and we don't even *realize* we can float or do something safe, so we end up exhausted from attempting to stay afloat and we can drown.

If we go to the car dealer and buy a brand new green Honda, suddenly it seems that everywhere we go people are driving green Hondas! It's not that they weren't there before; it is just that our subconscious mind hadn't been told they were important so we didn't consciously notice them.

This is the most interesting function of the subconscious mind because we can, through our own focused intent, change what our subconscious mind considers important or true, but this takes a lot of work and understanding of how to impact the conscious mind differently

When we make a decision to change some aspect of our lives, whether that be with regards to our health and wellness, our income, or our relationships, it can be hard to see how this change is going to occur. My suggestion is to take that first step, and it will become clear what path we need to travel.

For someone who has never experienced the power of their own subconscious mind, stepping out into the unknown can seem like a ludicrous idea. But what this concept really encourages us to do is to bring our desire to the full attention of our subconscious mind by taking that first step. Then we will be able to clearly see what needs to be done to get the next step, then the next, and so on. These things don't just appear. They already exist, but our subconscious mind didn't previously know to point them out to us, just like the green Hondas. Once we focus our attention and bring those ideas to our awareness, we will see the path ahead and discover the solutions that were always there, but were hidden from our conscious mind.

Intellectual Faculties

The vast majority of people live their lives allowing their environment and circumstances to control the way they think, feel, and act. The good news is that we have the power to take control of our thoughts independent of our environment. The best way to do this is through the development of the intellectual mind, or what we will call our intellectual faculties.

When we learn to effectively use our intellectual faculties, we can actively control our thoughts, which then control our feelings. These feelings move our body to a new and higher vibration, which ultimately affects the results we get in our lives. This accounts for why some people experience more of the results they want than others.

Napoleon Hill, in his book *Think and Grow Rich*, studied the richest, most powerful people in the world, and he found that "these people acquired this system of thinking and success in their lives, not because they had generalized knowledge, but because they had developed their intellectual faculties so they could create anything they wanted in their lives or its equivalent without violating the rights of other people." What he is saying is that the proper use of these intellectual faculties is really what allows us to control the way we think. When we learn to develop and use our intellectual faculties, we can really then begin to control our attitudes and ultimately the results we have in our lives.

Every person is born with intellectual faculties, and they need to be developed like we develop our physical muscles, by overcoming resistance. I like to call these "attitudinal muscles." Most of us give our conscious minds to our five senses rather than to the higher side of our intellectual nature because it's easier and requires little effort. This is natural human behavior—to take the path of least resistance. Eating a pizza is easier than running four miles. Watching a movie is easier than memorizing a poem. But what is easier is not always as fulfilling.

The development of these faculties will allow us to lead more fulfilling lives because we will be living our lives on purpose rather than floating through the days just accepting what occurs for us and having our thoughts go up and down like a roller coaster from all the stimuli of the senses. Learning to develop the intellectual factors, and thus learning to control the thoughts that enter our conscious minds, starts with being responsible for all of our emotions. When we are responsible for our emotions we can change them, but if we blame others for our emotions, then we will always feel like a victim. There is no personal power in being a victim. Responsibility leads to freedom.

So, let's take a look at these intellectual factors in more detail. These intellectual faculties are:

perception

will

imagination

memory

intuition

reason

Perception

Perception is how we view things in life—it is our version of reality. It is our perspective, our point of view. An example of this is if we look at a photograph or collage of many pictures together, we tend to focus on some things while we block out others. However, if another person is looking at the same photograph or collage, they will focus on different items than we did based on their knowledge and experiences.

If we showed that same collage to a group of people, then took it away after sixty seconds and asked them to write down a list of all the things that they saw, some things listed may be seen by part of the group but not all of them. Each list will be a little different. This is an example of the difference in perception from one person to another. We also place different meaning and significance on events in our lives, and we do this with perception. It is interesting that this shift in perception can also be experienced by siblings raised in the same environment and exposed to the same events. Even with many commonalities, there will still be a difference in how they each perceive the events.

*When we change the way we look at things, the
things we look at change.*

—Wayne Dyer

When information enters our conscious mind through the five senses, it is neither good nor bad. We use our perception, based on comparisons and context, to see it as positive or negative. Our perception is governed by the Law of Polarity, which states: for every up there is a down, for every in there is an out; in other words, there is no good without a little bad and no bad without a little good.

An example of people using perception to control their results in my field of dentistry is that some dentists have the perception that certain times of the year are better for the patients to have dental work. Some of my fellow dentists actually plan to be slower at certain times of the year based on their perception about patients or the past. This isn't necessarily the truth, but it is their perception. This belief influences their production during these times. Our perception that we will be slow at a certain time of the year will influence our thinking, and thus we are less productive during that time. It is like a self-fulfilling prophecy when those times actually are slow because of the perceptions held.

In any given situation there are always other viewpoints or sides to the story. They are neither good nor bad in and of themselves, but these answers are made so purely by our perspective of the situation. For example, if we have a minor accident on the way to work, we may perceive it to be horrible and a great inconvenience both to our finances and to our day. The other driver may be so grateful that her child was not injured, that she views the event with relief. Her perception is that it could have been so much worse. This is the power of perception.

Will

Will is our absolute ability to focus on one thing to the exclusion of all others. Will is what sees us through challenges. Another way of looking at will is to see it as persistence. Persistence and directed focus through all circumstances is a quality that makes the difference between the person who succeeds and the one who doesn't. Using our will keeps us on track to accomplish goals and to get past challenges or delays on the path to success. When we look at it from a medical view point, will is what keeps people alive through catastrophic accidents or illnesses when the odds are against them. It is what helps people heal more quickly. We even call this the will to live.

If a patient were to receive a diagnosis of cancer and the person chose to live, he would use his will to focus on health and well-being. He would use his will to focus on what he could do to heal and to feel better even during difficult treatments. This is using both will and perception to achieve a positive outcome. Using their will, patients can overcome all the overwhelming challenges that inevitably occur during treatment and wholly and completely be there to support their family and give and receive energy from others to continue healing. The will is so strong it can affect whether we live or die. We will frequently see a couple who have been married for decades die within months of one another—even if one spouse wasn't even sick. Without their life partner, they lose this intangible will to live and death soon follows.

My mother was sick most of my life. She had emphysema and chronic bronchitis from years of smoking—in fact, she smoked until the day she died. This condition is one that seriously debilitates the patient. She required oxygen on a continual basis and barely could take a step before she would be out of breath. My mother bounced from hospital bed to hospital bed throughout Connecticut, and various physicians attempted to treat her for not only her respiratory disease but also the addiction she developed to narcotic pain medication.

Emphysema is a condition which causes the lungs to lose their elasticity—the patient can't exhale the carbon dioxide efficiently—and this poison accumulates in the lungs and body. When this occurred, Mom would be placed on a respirator, where the lungs would be forced to empty the carbon dioxide, and her blood gasses would return to relatively healthy levels.

My mother had seven children and she loved them all, but I noticed that when her marriage finally fell apart and she was divorced from my father, she completely lost her desire to live, and within a year of the divorce my mother passed away. She had fought this terrible disease for years, but when her will was lost, her body simply would not fight anymore.

Bob Proctor says, "If we were to choose just one part of our personality to develop that would virtually guarantee our success, I'd like to suggest that we place persistence at the top of our list." Most people don't seem to realize that they have this great power within them if they choose to use it. Persistence is like running in a marathon. It is our will that keeps us going when our muscles ache and our body begs to quit. We keep pushing in spite of doubt and pain until we reach the finish line. Ralph Waldo Emerson said, "That which we give energy to will expand." What do we give energy to in our lives?

Persistence is a unique mental strength; a strength that is essential to combat the fierce power of the repeated rejections and numerous other obstacles that sit in waiting and are all part of winning in a fast-moving, ever-changing world.

—Bob Proctor

Imagination

This is our ability to build big, beautiful pictures in our minds. This is how we form clear pictures of what we want. Then, we use our will to hold them in our conscious mind as we work toward achieving what we want in life. Many of us imagine and dream of more money, better health, and a long life, but it is important to realize that we can choose positive or negative outcomes. Einstein had carved into his desk "imagination is more powerful than knowledge." If we can see it in our minds, then we can have it in our lives!

Everything in our home, the clothes we wear, the chair we sit on, and the pen we write with were nothing but a thought in someone's mind. The buildings in our community began with just a thought and a mental picture of what could be built. The people who decided to add buildings to the community sat down one day and wrote down their ideas and developed a picture of what it would look like in their minds! They then found contractors, architects, plumbers, electricians, carpenters, and masons to create these buildings in their physical forms. But it all started with a clear and vivid picture in their minds—in their imagination!

Everything starts with imagination. It is the proper use of this imagination that makes the difference in how healthy a life we live and the success we have in our lives. We can imagine great things happening to us, or we can imagine disaster. Unfortunately, many people focus on the worst possible case scenario for a situation. This is useful information, but should only be considered for a short time. Remember, what we focus on will expand!

For example, if a doctor understands the worst-case scenario, then the patient can be prepared for whatever may happen. But the key word here is understands vs. focuses. Focusing consumes us. Most people haven't used their imagination to its full capacity since they were children, but imagination can be developed. Children daydream about being in the mountains or on the beach, and they see themselves in a life that doesn't physically exist at the time. Imagination fosters reality. What are we imagining about our future health?

If Thomas Edison hadn't imagined the lightbulb, would electricity exist? Too often we see imagination as a negative and fanciful thing. Some would say that this doesn't get results and imagination is just a waste of time. This couldn't be farther from the truth, and we are usually told this by someone who has given up on imagination or by someone who has let negative thoughts come into their conscious mind and control their feelings, so we let their thoughts affect our thinking, influence our actions, and dull our imagination. However, by developing our imagination, we expand our ability to create whatever we want for our lives.

Memory

There are actually two aspects of memory to consider. First, there are our memories from life experiences that cover all the years from birth to the present. Second, there is the act of remembering or recalling information.

The power of memory is that we have the ability to choose what we want to remember. For example, very few women choose to remember the pain of childbirth because we focus on and remember the joy we felt when the baby was put in our arms the first time. We choose to forget the awkwardness of braces as teenagers and remember the confidence we gained from a wonderful smile. What do we remember as we think back on our childhood? We can choose to remember all of our triumphs and all the praise we have received to make us feel great. Sometimes people forget that they can make the choice to remember the good things and experiences they've had, and this is a great way to get into a positive mental state.

Unfortunately, many people remember only the failures, all the times they have fallen and the criticism received. We take all these collective memories about why we are no good or unable to achieve what we want. Too often, we drag our past into our future. It's like carrying around a backpack full of heavy rocks. Each one of the rocks represents a negative belief or thought that we hold about ourselves. For some reason, we think we have to keep carrying it around everywhere we go, and it just gets heavier and heavier as the years pass. Most of us don't even realize that we are carrying this extra load because we are so used to it that we actually think it is part of us, but in fact, if we were able to rid ourselves of these limiting beliefs, we would be much lighter and feel more freedom in all aspects of our lives.

Even in old age we hear a little voice in our head saying, "You are no good at math," or "Your life didn't amount to much." Why do we do this? We have already paid for these things in our past. Why do we feel we need to continue to pay for them? When working toward achieving our dream it is critical to remember the successes. It is important to develop the positive memories and let the negative ones go. What is that little voice saying in your head?

When we let go of the negative beliefs and thoughts, then our backpack of rocks gets lighter. Our positive beliefs and thoughts that replace the negative ones are as light as balloons. After a while, we aren't carrying a heavy backpack and we feel good about ourselves and our dreams. This has positive physical outcomes for us. We feel less stressed, and we are able to relax more. This will manifest differently for each person, but in general, if we are able to let go of the negative past and focus on our dreams we tend to feel better physically.

We need to let our memories support our dreams! Put the failures where they belong—in the past! Mahareshi Mahesh Yogi, the person who introduced Transcendental Meditation to the West, said, "I use my memory, but I don't allow my memories to use me."

Intuition

If prayer is us talking to God,
intuition is God talking to us.

—Wayne Dyer

Intuition is our ability to pick up the energy from someone else. Have you ever walked into a room and sensed the energy there? This is an example of our intuition picking up the vibration of the people in the room, and it usually happens on a very subconscious level. We just feel it.

Bob Proctor teaches in his *You Were Born Rich* course that in the early 1930s, scientists invented a form of photography that could take a specialized picture that allows us to see energy leaving the body. These frequencies, or energy auras, project our energy out to others and attracts those with similar energy. We can intuitively sense that energy from others. If we are expressing lack, anger, or limitations, then we are sending out the energy of doubt and negativity.

Intuition is also how we become consciously aware of ideas. It is what is commonly referred to as the sixth sense or a hunch. It works with our subconscious mind to give out information and the feeling of direction. If we have an intuitive sense about something, then ask, "If I act on this idea, will it bring me closer to my goal?" We wouldn't have desired it if we couldn't do it! If this idea will bring us closer to our dream, then act on it. We need to develop our intuition and learn to trust it.

Reason

Reasoning is our ability to think and choose. When an idea enters our conscious mind, we have the ability to process the information and decide if it is something we are going to act on or not. We can gather independent facts and create our own conclusion. We can also have a conclusion in our mind, and then we can go out and find the facts to support this conclusion.

Problems or circumstances require reasoning so that we can understand the relationships between facts. Our mind takes all these different facts and links them together like a chain, sees how they are related, and then makes sense of it. Reasoning is similar to logical thinking and is made up of sequential thinking patterns. This process takes important ideas, facts, and information we gather through our five senses. Then, our mind works through that information and gives us the solution to our problem or situation. Reasoning is our logical side of the mind. It is deductive in nature while imagination is inductive.

Proper use of these intellectual faculties, blended with our thoughts, allows us to affect how we feel. In turn, our feelings affect what kind of vibration we are sending out into the universe. That negative or positive energy ultimately affects all we attract in our lives. The first step is to develop an awareness and then practice using the intellectual faculties. By doing this, we not only gain control of our intellectual mind, but we can directly affect our subconscious mind, feelings, and ultimately our actions. When we allow these intellectual faculties to govern our thoughts, this allows us to be proactive as opposed to living in reaction mode. We can achieve anything we want when we are proactive, but when we are reactionary, we lose our power and fall into the victim trap.

When we talk about awareness, we are talking about self-awareness. To be clear about the difference between awareness and self-awareness we should look at their definitions. According to the *Encarta World English Dictionary*, awareness is defined as "knowing something because we have observed it or someone has told us about it." It is a matter of noticing or realizing that something exists. As we study, react, and speak to experts, we learn and thus increase our awareness about this topic. Self-awareness is defined as having a balanced and honest view of our own personality, and this can be extremely challenging.

To be aware that there is a mind-body connection is very important as it relates to others, but to be aware of how it personally manifests in our own lives is to be self-aware. The importance of becoming self-aware is the first step in this path of living a life that we can fully enjoy. Awareness is a part of the creative process of our lives. The more self-aware we are, the more we develop our intuition, the more we will be able to access our true potential when problems arise.

Once we understand ourselves better, we will have the opportunity to change and create the lives we want. Increased self-awareness requires seriously looking at ourselves and discovering blind spots. This occurs through coaching and listening to others we trust. Once we are aware of our blind spots, we can then apply the principles in this book to change our thoughts, change our feelings, and ultimately change our actions and results.

Let us not look back in anger, nor forward in fear, but around in awareness.

—James Thurber

For some, the concept of self-awareness and self-improvement is a new idea. I believe it is one of the most important pieces of the puzzle that builds a healthy self-esteem, confidence, and a healthy body. We have to know ourselves first in order to make changes. Some of the areas included in becoming self-aware and really knowing ourselves are discovered by asking the following questions:

Do we know what our strengths and weaknesses are?

What are our desires?

What do we want in life?

What motivates us?

What makes us feel sad?

What makes us feel happy?

Is there something that we want to change about ourselves already?

What have we achieved so far in our life?

What do we want to achieve?

What seems to be stopping us from achieving our goals?

What beliefs do we hold?

What values are important to us?

When answering these questions, we are assessing our thoughts, feelings, and emotions. We might even sit down with someone we love and trust and review them and take note if our answers are positive or negative. This is very indicative of our emotional state. Let's take a moment and apply this to our health. Are we aware of the physical signals that our body sends to us to let us know if something is wrong? Do we ignore them? Are we realistic about our health and fitness?

What we are striving for is an understanding of self that allows us to live in harmony physically, spiritually, and mentally. Becoming more self-aware will also assist us in maintaining a healthy life. We'll be more in tune with our body and the messages it sends us. In the same way, if we have had a medical procedure or have been sick, then we recover much more quickly and are more in tune with the changes brought about by our own healing. Our body has an incredible ability to heal, but we must be in a relaxed state to allow this to occur.

I don't treat patients with life-threatening problems as a periodontist, but I do see many manifestations of fear and stress. Grace is a woman in her early 50s who came to me with bleeding and inflamed gums. She was afraid. She was going to lose her teeth, but she was too afraid to come in to see me. This had gone on for a long time, and Grace neither sought care nor practiced good dental hygiene because she was allowing fear to guide her.

As we worked with her to do the required procedures to get her mouth healthy she had some major doubts and was very fearful. I spent time discussing how positive attitudes and beliefs would affect her healing process. We built her confidence and knowledge, and then we took steps to find out what thoughts or beliefs she was holding about herself that kept her from feeling like she could be completely healthy.

Through talking with this patient I found out that she had a reoccurring dream for years that all of her teeth fell out. That thought had come from deep in her subconscious mind and only surfaced in her dreams. It turns out that as a small child she was around great-aunts, great-uncles, and grandparents who all had dentures. She heard many stories from her mother about dental problems that develop with everyone as they get older.

As a child she had trouble with her baby teeth and had several extracted. When her permanent teeth came in, they were very crowded. As a teenager she went through braces and additional extractions. Some of the experiences had been difficult for her, and all this information was stored away in her subconscious mind with what she thought she knew about getting older. She became fearful of going to the dentist and tried to ignore her body's messages until she couldn't ignore them anymore.

We were able to work through her feelings, and she realized that the beliefs she had were not really related to her dental reality at all. She was not at all in danger of losing her teeth. She simply needed to take better care of her dental hygiene. We discussed the treatment plan thoroughly, and she began practicing visualization of the results she wanted. She went on to smile with confidence, and she learned to apply these principles not only to help with her dental fear but also to help her overcome other fears as well. Her self-image improved, and her sense of self-value increased.

As happened with my patient, awareness is the first step on the way to healing one's body, and making changes about the beliefs we may have learned as a child are critical in this process. Our awareness allows us to change the way we think and ultimately change our results. We alter the body's new vibration, and this enhances our efforts. The vibration we are in will also attract more of the same types of energy toward us. If we choose to develop and use the intellectual faculties in a more positive way, we can change our vibration and change the energy attracted to us. We can therefore use our thoughts to change anything we want in our lives.

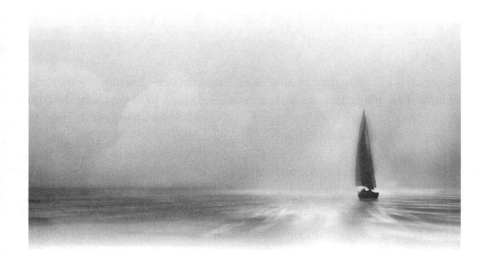

Chapter Four

—Fear—

Change your beliefs and you change your behavior.
Change your behaviors and you change your results.
Change your results and you change your life.

—Lisa Jimenez, from her book *Conquer Fear*

Chapter Four

Jenny can't decide what the spot is on her arm. She's heard disheartening stories of people getting rashes and spots and going in to get them checked out only to discover they are cancer. She even knows a few friends this has happened to, but Jenny thinks cancer can't happen to her. It happens to everyone else, but not her. She thinks that if she ignores it, the mark will go away, like a bruise or blemish.

So Jenny lets it go. She puts it out of her mind until a friend finally asks about it. Jenny has noticed that it has grown and changed and darkened in color, but the fear that it might actually be something serious has turned her awareness into denial.

It's nothing, she says to her friend. I've had this for awhile now. Really, it's fine.

A month goes by and still she can't put the mark out of her head. It can't be cancer, she thinks. I have a husband, a family, I'm a mother. I can't get cancer. Unfortunately, Jenny's fear has left her mentally debilitated. Her anxiety had grown to the point that she wouldn't go for any check up. When her husband finally convinced her go in to check on the spot, the doctor suggested a comprehensive examination, and after some initial hesitation, Jenny finally agreed.

A week later the biopsy on the spot comes back negative, but the lump in her breast, the one that she reluctantly had checked out, did not. Because Jenny allowed fear to take control of her decisions, ultimately her health was put at risk. According to the Law of Attraction, whatever we focus on, we attract. It really is about our awareness level. We become more aware, and therefore we notice or focus on something. Jenny brought the fear of cancer and poor health into her life. She focused on it, worried about it, and avoided steps that could have allowed her to get treatment earlier and therefore would have prevented it from spreading. Many people fear health problems and disease. This could be due to past experiences with loved ones who were ill, or it could be true or imagined fear about their mortality. While health concerns are normal, irrational fear and obsession around them is not.

There are different ways to define fear. First, it is an emotion that is felt strongly in anticipation of some kind of pain or danger. This kind of fear will trigger our fight or flight reflex. Adrenaline pumps into our body, and we can run faster and jump higher than usual to get away from the source of our fear. This helps us function better for the short term. Another way to define fear is that it can be more of an ongoing anxious feeling, which is very unhealthy over the long term. Some would describe this emotion as worry or excessive stress. It is frequently felt by people with financial problems, relationship issues, and health concerns, but it is important to realize that fear can be very detrimental to our health.

I've heard it said that fear is interesting because it is entirely a perception of the mind. Right now we might be healthy and strong. But when we think about events of the past, or what might happen in the future, we can allow fear to completely overwhelm us. This often happens when, like Jenny, we see a small sign that triggers our emotional response. It could be a small spot on the arm that gives us a fear of cancer, a momentary lapse in thought that causes us to fear Alzheimer's disease, or a slight chest pain that convinces us that a heart attack is unavoidable. All of these symptoms by themselves could easily be nothing at all, or they may be the early signs of something more dangerous developing. But because we let fear escalate, we bring on more problems and often refuse to find solutions in the earliest stages when the symptoms can be simply taken care of or eliminated.

The Impact of Fear on our Health

When a fear becomes a phobia, the effects can be seen in our health. A patient of mine, we'll call her Betty, came to me with a rather unusual question for a periodontist. I hadn't seen her in awhile, but when she finally came in she said she'd heard that I was well-researched in the philosophy of the mind controlling how the body responds as it relates to good health or poor health, and she hoped that I'd be able to help. Betty, who was 21, told me that her fear of social situations had become quite debilitating; even coming in to talk to me was extremely difficult. Ever since high school, she said, her fear and anxiety had left her socially isolated.

"I was unable to go to my prom because the anxiety got to be too much; even going out to movies and dinner was hard. I had to excuse myself from the table throughout the night and sit in the bathroom in one of the stalls. My sweating got out of control. My shirt would literally be drenched in sweat."

Betty had headaches, stomach aches, and terrible insomnia. She wept in my office. She hadn't been able to tell anyone of her fears. She felt alone. Through the tears, she went on to say that it had gotten to the point that even in her own home she felt scared and anxious, yet she didn't know why. The fear had grown to such proportions that she was a prisoner in her own home.

Betty felt helpless to change things, so I encouraged her to see that the first step was the understanding that we all choose our thoughts. We must choose to change our thoughts and change our lives. That doesn't mean it's easy—in fact, it can be the hardest thing we have ever done in our lives. We all create a comfort zone, and even if that comfort zone limits our lives we still find it easier to stay within the walls of our own creation than choose to change. However, it is this power to choose that really gives us our freedom to heal.

Betty had used this fear to convince herself that she was hopeless, when it was the farthest thing from the truth. Knowing we are in control is very empowering, but it involves accepting responsibility for our current situation. Because Betty constantly allowed herself to be in a fearful and negative state of mind, she attracted more fear and negativity into her life.

The good news is that she could choose differently—and she did. It happened slowly over time as she forced herself into social situations to confront her fears, and soon they diminished to allow her to lead a much more normal life. She used visualization to imagine herself in the situation relaxed and comfortable, and to her excitement that's exactly what happened. As I expected, she arrived back in my office a few months later saying she still had a way to go, but that her life had completely changed since she changed her thoughts. She felt wonderful and was able to go out with friends and even date a little. Better yet, she was sharing what she had learned with others so they too could move through their fears, choose to change their thoughts, and live a more healthy, happy life.

The Terror Barrier

Even if you have not heard of the term terror barrier, I am sure you have experienced at least once or twice in life. It is that point we reach when we feel that we cannot push through our fears and move forward. The fear becomes an insurmountable obstacle that we see no way around or through. In short, we're stuck. This is a situation in which we have a new thought clashing with our old limiting beliefs in our subconscious mind. The clash between the new thought and old belief causes us to literally freeze. This is a critical point in moving forward with our new idea. Our old conditioning can be very powerful, and it will challenge new ideas. If we are unaware of this we will usually give the old results. If we are aware that this is occurring we can push through this fear called the terror barrier, and we can move into new thinking. We can create new beliefs and paradigms, and ultimately we will see the new, better results.

I experienced the terror barrier when I was first learning surgical procedures and techniques. There had to be a first time that I held a scalpel and faced my first patient. I have to say, I was extremely fearful. My old conditioning told me that I couldn't do the procedure, and even though I had learned how to perform surgery and I felt completely confident that I could do the procedure, I was still really scared. Eventually, of course, I did overcome that fear, but it took some time and a lot of visualization. What old conditioning or old beliefs are holding you back?

Our fears can feel controlling and oppressive. They seem to control us instead of us controlling them. Fear can literally stop us in our tracks and keep us from progressing toward what we really want. We believe that we cannot pass that imaginary line whether it is starting a new business, committing to a relationship, or having that long-awaited physical examination. It is like a threshold we cannot bring ourselves to cross. Everyone responds differently to this, but some may physically feel shaky, break out in a cold sweat, feel their heart slamming in their chest and their mouth go dry, while others may just feel completely unsure or just plain scared. Since we believe we cannot go any further, our perception becomes our reality.

Where does this barrier come from? We all have ideas that are actually limiting beliefs that we have acquired from others in our lives as we grew up. They may include things such as "Money doesn't grow on trees," or with regards to our health, "Cancer is a killer," or "Twenty pounds overweight means 20 years off our life," or even, "If we don't exercise, we're a ticking time bomb." We also acquire beliefs from our own experiences in our past.

These statements and the consequent embedded paradigms have taken up permanent residence in our mind. However, there is a way to dislodge them and change them. In essence, we can break through that terror barrier no matter how long we've had it or how well established it is. It is all about awareness and changing our thoughts. We need to be aware that each time we attempt to make a major move or change in our lives we **will** have to face this terror barrier. When we know what to expect, then we can simply acknowledge that our fear has resurfaced, but we don't have to allow it to stop us. We are strong and will move through our fear.

However, it takes a fair amount of discipline to choose to change, and just because we choose it once doesn't mean that we will be strong enough to push through this terror barrier time and time again. Each day we must choose again the thoughts we want. This is why it is so easy to slide back into our old habits and let fear overwhelm us. If we are not vigilant in our awareness, then we will tend to give into the fear and we're right back where we were in our old thoughts and beliefs. It is not uncommon to take three steps forward and two steps back—repeatedly. Old ideas and habits don't just disappear. We must be persistent to put those old ways out of our life time and again.

Bulldozing through the terror barrier is one way to get through it. We do not stop for anything. The threshold is there, but we do not stop and wait; we force ourselves to make a decision to proceed. We just keep going, in spite of our feelings and in spite of our intense fear. The realization that we survived crashing through the barrier will encourage us to do it again the next time it rears its ugly head. Make the decision ahead of time to keep going and we will not hesitate to move forward. Refuse to permit emotions and fear of the unknown to control us. Cross the threshold to the future!

You gain strength, courage, and confidence from every experience in which you really stop to look fear on the face. You must do the thing you think you cannot do.

—Eleanor Roosevelt

Fear of Failure

Who hasn't been afraid to fail? Not only do self-limiting beliefs create irrational fear, but they also place limitations on our lives because we believe certain things about ourselves and our abilities. These beliefs are largely unconscious and may be completely unfounded, for example beliefs like: I am overweight, there's no way anyone will love me; or, I am not lucky, it won't happen to me, it never does; or possibly, I won't get the job, so I'm not even going to try. The fact that someone is overweight has no relation to love. Similarly, bad luck has no determination whether or not someone gets a better job. In fact, I love the saying, "Luck is really God being anonymous!" Yet we frequently connect these ideas in our mind, not even stopping to consider if they are really true or not.

Much like fear, limitations are a perception of the mind. In reality, we have no limitations and can do anything if we put our minds to it. Determination always finds a way around obstacles. Our thoughts and beliefs color our vision and perception of the world. They determine our actions or inactions. Thoughts affect feelings. Feelings affect behavior. Behavior produces results, negative or positive. It all begins with our thoughts, and, remembering back to the conscious mind that we discussed earlier, we have to accept our thoughts in order for them to move into our subconscious mind where they become beliefs.

Consider that whatever we believe becomes our reality. We do not believe what we see; rather, we see what we already believe. For this reason, two people facing the same situation may interpret it differently, act according to their different beliefs, and experience different outcomes.

Self-limiting beliefs are roadblocks to our progress, brakes causing us to lose momentum and ultimately stop. We pretend we are moving forward, tricking our mind into believing there is forward motion, when in reality we're going backward. Attempting to move toward the positive when we have negative programming is like expecting a photocopy to be different from the original. We've got to work on the original copy first, change the blueprint, and rework the thoughts in the conscious mind.

Our thoughts and beliefs directly cause our actions, which show up as our existence, our lives. We cannot move beyond them without changing our thoughts first. To get out of the never ending cycle of acting positive but believing negative, we've got to identify these negative thoughts and self-limiting fears and eliminate them, consciously and consistently. Sometimes the struggle will last longer than we anticipate, but it's a struggle that we can and will win each time. This is when we need to tap into the intellectual faculty we call will.

In order to make these changes, we first have to identify our self-limiting beliefs and write them down. To find them in our own life, we can look at any area where we've experienced failure, any situation we frequently avoid, or any event that elicits an emotional response from us. We might see a basketball court and remember the time we were cut from the team in high school. Or we might see a movie and be taken back to a relationship that ended after leaving a theater. We may feel anger over a friend who hurt us. Memories can be triggered by a number of things. And all these memories, which reside in the subconscious mind, will automatically cause us to react in certain ways based on these past experiences unless we understand this process and change our conscious thoughts.

Once we have identified our own self-limiting beliefs, these fears must be challenged every time they enter our mind. We must consciously reject any thought or suggestion of failure. We have limitless potential and personal power, and this power is within us right now. We can tap into our power to choose, and all that hinders us from becoming whatever we want in our lives can be changed. When fear is starved of attention, when it's forgotten, it's like a scavenger that can no longer find food. That fear will drift away because it knows it cannot survive. Change our awareness and focus on thoughts in harmony with our goals and dreams, and we will attract more of this into our lives.

Jim Rohn says it aptly: "You cannot take the mild approach to the weeds in your mental garden. You have got to hate weeds enough to kill them. Weeds are not something you handle; weeds are something you devastate." You must encourage the positive and annihilate the negative thoughts that enter your mind. Let in and nurture only those that support your dreams and move you toward your goals.

Overcoming Our Fears

A colleague of mine, a therapist dealing with different anxiety disorders, told me that she encourages her patients to write down on paper their fears, their concerns, and their limitations so they can go back and objectively look at what they once thought was a realistic ideology. They then write the opposite of those fears and express the outcome they want. These become the ideas that they were to focus on every day. By searching for these alternative thoughts, letting these positive thoughts into their conscious minds, her clients are able to take action, step by step, and avoid things that were previously done with negative thoughts in mind.

The most comforting aspect of this idea is that after realizing what needs to happen, what thoughts the patients need to focus on, and which ones they release from thought, the patients understand that they are not alone. That comfort itself is often enough to let go of the anxiety.

A better way to deal with self-limiting thoughts is to prevent them from entering our conscious mind in the first place. Remember, we choose all the thoughts entering our conscious mind and we cannot develop a belief unless we have accepted it as a thought first. This is when we need to develop our intellectual faculties so we can choose powerfully to accept only the thoughts that forward us toward our goals and dreams. If we learn to develop our ability to do this powerfully and reject harmful thoughts, we will be well on our way to living a happy, healthy, prosperous life.

One of the most interesting concepts of shifting to a positive attitude is to understand the role of failure. This may sound contradictory, but the Law of Polarity states that we can't have success without failure. The real understanding is in viewing failure as feedback rather than an indictment of us as people. Just because we fail is no reason to stop or give up. Achievers keep working and focusing on the end results they want, and they move through their fear into success.

The Wright Brothers, Thomas Edison, and Martin Luther King Jr. all had failed at one time in their lives—in fact, they all failed repeatedly. Persistence (will) and perception (i.e., the ability to admit and nurture the positive aspects of those previous failures) led them to success. We never would have flown if the Wright brothers had given up when their first flying machine went down. We might still be in the dark if Thomas Edison had believed what his teachers said about his lack of initiative and intellect, and we all would be in a very different place if Martin Luther Jr. hadn't kept pushing for change.

Once we make the decision to succeed, there is no going back. We can move only forward. The bridges of our negativity must be burned. Success and failure are polar opposites. We can't experience one without experiencing the other, but we can have both at the same time. My suggestion is to set a goal of happiness and freedom; set a goal worth failing for. And as John Maxwell would say, "Make it big enough that it is just worth failing for and then fail forward."

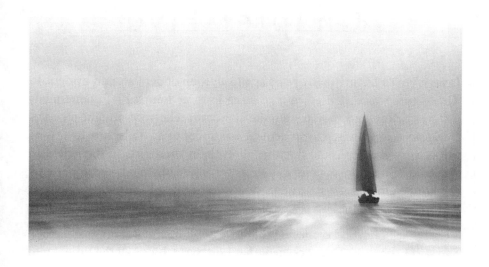

Chapter Five

—Courage—

*You can conquer almost any fear if you will make up
your mind to do so. For remember, fear doesn't exist
anywhere except in the mind.*

—Dale Carnegie

Chapter Five

I was giving a lecture many years ago to a group of dentists and hygienists. The lecture was supposed to take place in three hours. I had done many lectures before and they were quite standard, relatively straight forward. But instead of speaking to students, I was about to give a lecture to a room full of very accomplished doctors, all of them specialists in their fields. I was talking with my daughter as I was getting ready to go, and apparently she knew something was wrong. She looked at me and asked if something was wrong, and I told her, "Nothing."

"Really," she said. So I confessed that I was a bit nervous about this lecture. She said I shouldn't be concerned; that I do these things all the time. I told her that it was a bit different this time.

"Why?" she asked. And then she said something incredible, something I can't believe came out of her mouth. "Mom, you can't be brave if you're never scared."

I looked at her, this little girl, her head only coming to my waist, and I thought, she's right. She's absolutely right. How can there be bravery without fear? How can courage exist if there is no fear? Again, the Law of Polarity states that for everything there is an opposite. Courage is the opposite of fear, and without one there cannot be the other.

When we hear the word "courage," I am sure each of us can think of someone we have known or a person in the public eye who has done something courageous. We think of soldiers, firefighters, police officers, and people in our communities who make a difference. We think about rescuers that gave their all on 9/11. We love to hear about the courage of others. We read books and watch movies about brave deeds. Courage can be defined as bravery, will, fortitude, audacity, gallantry, intrepidity. Courage is the ability to confront fears, danger, take risks, go through pain, uncertainty, and intimidation. Courage is listening to greater good. Moral courage is when someone takes the correct stand and does the right thing in spite of popular opinion or opposition, challenges or discouragement. For our focus, we are looking at physical courage in the face of self-limiting beliefs, medical conditions, physical pain, hardship, and even the threat of death through disease.

Why are some people more courageous than others? The truth is, we all have the same potential of exhibiting certain behaviors. We make the mistake of thinking courage is for the few and the strong, that we are too old, or too young, but the truth is that courage can exist in every background.

For example: I happened to catch the opening ceremonies of the Olympics in Beijing when the giant Yao Ming walked out holding the Chinese flag. There was a tiny little boy walking next to him, and he literally almost looked fake next to Yao; he almost looked like a doll. His hand disappeared as Yao's hand held onto it. The announcer came on to say that this little boy, Lin Hao, a survivor of the devastating May 13 earthquake, saved two of his fellow students. Lin Hao was only nine years old.

When asked by the BBC what happened, the tiny Lin Hao said, "The corridor collapsed as I was walking. Two of my classmates were trapped beside me. I tried as hard as I could to climb out, and after I had climbed out I pulled a classmate out." The classmate was unconscious. And then to make things even more remarkable, Lin Hao went back in for another classmate.

We could share stories for a thousand pages about great deeds and heroic men and women, but what I want to stress here is that we—yes, we—have tremendous courage within us. It doesn't need to be something as dramatic as saving lives or helping victims in natural disasters. Courage doesn't hold one face.

During the Fourth of July parade I was sitting next to a boy who was about eleven years old. He was smiling the whole time. He spoke in a different accent. I overheard someone ask where they were from, and the boy's older brother or father, I couldn't tell which, said Siberia. God, I thought, no wonder the little guy's smiling; he can wear shorts here!

In his hands was a bag. The bag was filled with candy thrown out during the parade. The little boy couldn't speak English well and leaned over and asked his brother a question in Russian. The brother answered him, and the little boy leaned over to the young girl who was sitting next to him and said in broken English, "I want share. You share? This too much for one person."

I was totally floored. What kind of kid says that? I was overcome with emotion. His soft voice asking a stranger to share his candy with him because it was too much for him alone. I realized this was a different kind of courage all together. Not one of heroism or bravery, but courage to be himself, courage to commit to love and kindness.

The first step to knowing how to become courageous is to know where courage originates. It is not a clear-cut formula that shows us where we can find courage. However, it begins with small things. Courage is linked with our feelings and emotions about our own experiences and others we have seen. After 9/11, the question was asked over and over: why would someone run into a disintegrating building to save someone they do not even know when everything in us instinctively tells us to run in the other direction? Why would a nine-year-old child go back into a crumbling school to pull out two other students? Why would a boy from Siberia be so intuitively selfless? There is a risk involved anytime we decide to take a stand or face a challenge, no matter how small or large it may be. I believe it has to do with a positive self-image and a confidence in ourselves that we overcome. When Lin Hao was asked why he did what he did, he said, "I was the class leader and hall monitor that day." He embodied positive thoughts and then passed that on to others.

Most people have a fear of public speaking, yet the one who is determined will do it through their fear. It is not a matter of being fearless; it is a matter of being aware of our fears and functioning through them. Even though this is true, taking a risk in the face of adversity appears to be a huge stumbling block for most people. I suggest that a major reason for this lack of courage is based on people not wanting to see or sense reality. Courage starts when each of us decides we want to open our eyes and willingly examine ourselves and our world. We must allow ourselves to face the truth.

We've talked a lot about positive mental attitude and positive thinking as tools to good health and physical fitness, but that is only part of the answer, although it is a great foundation to build on. However, things do not change unless we are willing to listen to our own intuition. The next step is to take action to bring those positive ideas to fruition.

Hopefully as a result of reading this book, you have done some reflecting on yourself—your beliefs, thought patterns, and behaviors. I encourage you to keep moving forward. You already have the courage to go the next step, and you have come a long way from when we started this journey. I am sure that we can think of things we want to change about ourselves, and this can lead us to change the entire world around us. Start on the inside and work out. Gandhi once said, "We must be the change we want to see in the world."

Fear and love seem to be a part of our motivation to develop and use courage. As stated in the previous chapter, fear can be a great motivator. If we are more afraid to let things stay the way they are than we are to move forward to the unknown, we usually stay stuck in sickness and sadness.

Love is a factor in building courage because it is a matter of doing something to make our situation better because we love our children and family—and ourselves. That love for others encourages us to act courageously and to find the strength that it takes to see something all the way through to the end. Eleanor Roosevelt called it finding strength and stamina "to do the thing we think we cannot do." In the process, we will meet resistance, and this is expected. It can be internal or external resistance. However, stick with it and we will succeed. Believe we can accomplish our goals; we can lead a healthy and balanced life.

The Relationship Between Courage and Our Health

It takes courage to face the truth and then find a solution to health challenges. Our personal courage will give us what we need to face the consequences and do what needs to be done to restore our health.

Our attitude influences how we feel. A false belief that we catch everything that goes around during the winter sets us up for getting sick repeatedly during the cold months. However, if we are willing to recognize these old beliefs, then we can reflect on why we think this way. Were we told we were sickly as a child? Did we have asthma when growing up, but grow out of it as an adult? Yet, we are still having attacks periodically in the cold months. When we tell ourselves , "I'm always getting sick," then we will always get sick. When we hear rumors or see coworkers coming down with colds and we automatically think, "Shoot, I'm going to get sick now," then we will! That which we think about we become. The mind is able to process this negative feeling and manifest it into a sickness.

If we hear the same news about a cold circulating and think, "All right, I better wash my hands more often, and I think I will get to bed earlier tonight," we are instilling the mind-set and positive thought, and therefore we will experience better health. Be careful what we think about! Remember our subconscious minds cannot differentiate between real and imagined.

A patient of mine told me about his experience that would seem by conventional standards to be a contradiction. Terry is a handsome man, tall and blond, very Scandinavian looking, is in his mid-60s, and as a child had all of the childhood diseases that were around—chicken pox, measles, mumps, strep throat, tonsillitis, and of course seasonal colds and flu. He spent a lot of time in bed.

"That was the worst," he said. "Being in bed all day. I could hear the kids playing out on the street, their laughing and shouting. I could hear them running on the pavement, the bouncing of basketballs, those quick little pops, you know, when we put baseball cards in our spokes? It was terrible. I'd lay there all day and listen to this."

In elementary school, he spent two or three years with urinary infection problems. He had a few accidents on his bike and falls from trees, but the only injury was a broken arm. He loved sports and had a few minor injuries over the years. He had a few dental problems with cavities, and he needed braces in his early teens. All in all he did great through all of these challenges, until he contracted pneumonia at age fourteen. The doctor told his parents that he would always have to be careful, and his mother interpreted this to mean that he should never swim in cold water. He could get pneumonia again if he was not careful. To this day his mother thinks he shouldn't go into a lake or swim in the ocean. With a past like this, we can't help but think Terry must consider himself a sick person. However, Terry has always considered himself a healthy person.

"That was the whole crazy part about this all. In my head I saw myself as healthy. I played football in the fall, hockey in the winter, track in the spring. When I wasn't in bed sick, I'd be running through the neighborhood with the other kids, outrunning them even, until the sun went down and our mothers called us in. I wasn't an unhealthy person. And it always made me mad when I'd hear people say that I was sick. Poor Terry this, and poor Terry that. There was nothing poor about me. I didn't need anyone's pity. I was healthy; I just had a few infections every now and again."

Terry didn't pay any attention to other people. He believed that he was healthy, and one day he made a resolution to never be bedridden again.

"I was tired of it—tired of people limiting me, making my mind up for me. Their constant conversation about my illnesses was influencing my health. I was continuing to get sick. Maybe they were right, I thought. I didn't want to spend anymore of my childhood in bed. I didn't want to hear the kids playing outside without me. So I said, "This is the last day I'm going to spend in bed." I will never forget what happened next. The next morning I woke up and got out of bed. My head hurt like crazy and I was dizzy and my legs shook a little, but I left the bed and walked outside." Terry told me, "I had to sit down on the front steps for awhile to catch my breath, but I left my bed. My mom came out with this worried look on her face, telling me I was in no shape to be up, and I was too sick to be out of bed. I don't know what it was or why I did it, but when I looked up at my mom and thought of going back to bed and missing out on what all the other kids were doing, I started to cry. I told her, 'I'm sick of being in bed. I'm sick of being a kid in bed. I don't want to be a kid in bed anymore.' My mom started to cry too. She hugged me and told me to at least wear a sweater—giving her blessing to my recovery.

"And that was it. That was the last time I was ever bedridden. When I made the decision to get out of bed and stop wasting my life, my health changed. I don't know if I outgrew some childhood illness thing or what, but since then I have been incredibly healthy. I might get a cold every couple of years, but nothing big, nothing that really hinders me. I feel like when I made that choice to leave my bed; that was the bravest thing I have ever done." He laughed again. "That and having children."

Terry believes that it was his courage that helped him to become healthy and live the life he wanted to live. Courage doesn't have to be running into a collapsing building or throwing ourselves in front of a car to save someone. Courage has many facets, many faces, and can be as simple as getting out of bed when we don't feel like we can.

Mary's story:

Mary is now in her late 70s and suffered a massive heart attack at age 65. It came as a complete surprise to her family and to her. As far as she knew she did not have heart disease in her family, but her husband did, and she had always been concerned that he might have a heart attack. I believe this focus was at least part of the reason it happened to her. She was obsessed with what they should eat and worried all the time about his possible heart attack. She underwent bypass surgery and recovered over several months because she believed it was not her time to go yet. It was courageous for her to make the decision to have a quadruple bypass, but she believed she would be fine and that she had many more years ahead of her.

Honest courage is not the omission of fear, but the zeal to continue in spite of it.

—Marianna Ruiz

Many people know Louise Hay and her books on metaphysics—the role of our beliefs and how we think in relationship to our health. Metaphysics, according to the *Encarta World English Dictionary* is "a philosophy that is concerned with the study of the nature of being and beings, existence, time, and space, and causality." As noted in her book, *Heal Your Body*, Louise Hay overcame many obstacles in both her life as a child and adult when she started working on her own personal and spiritual growth. She had to recreate the way she thought and what she believed about herself.

Hay was enjoying her personal life and her work. She spent her time speaking, writing, and working with clients to improve their self-concepts, beliefs, and health. Then, she was diagnosed with cancer. She considered her background of being raped at five years old and having been a battered child and how those experiences affected her thoughts over the years. She realized that these thoughts had manifested within her as cervical cancer. At first she panicked. The news of such an illness is devastating. But a solid mental awareness told her to rely on what she knew and how she had helped her own clients. She knew that mental healing worked, and she had a chance to prove it to herself. Louise realized that her cancer was the result of her deep resentment for what she'd been through. Because she had never gotten rid of her anger and resentment, her resentment was buried for years. She realized that if she was going to survive the cancer, then she had a lot of personal work to do.

Louise Hay spent most of her childhood enduring hard labor, as well as physical and sexual abuse, and her self-esteem was low. It had taken years for her to develop higher expectations for herself. During this time of growth, she realized that the behavior patterns that she had in her home were also reflected in what she did in the outside world. She felt like she couldn't learn enough and couldn't read enough. She had a voracious appetite for more knowledge. Hay learned everything she could about metaphysics and healing. This was the turning point in her life.

After her cancer diagnosis, Louise Hay knew that she had to make a decision about having surgery to take out the cancer growth. Louise realized that she also had to get rid of any negative feelings or doubts about her recovery. She needed to change her mental pattern in order to keep the cancer from coming back. She believed that she could clear up the thought patterns that she believed had created her cancer. She didn't think she needed an operation. She finally convinced her doctors to give her three months. She needed the time to have the money to pay for the operation. However, she also wanted to give herself a chance to heal the cancer.

She took complete responsibility for her healing. She investigated and read about alternative methods of healing. She went to health food stores and bought books about cancer. She read everything on the subject at the library. Louise tried reflexology and colon therapy. Sitting in the back of a lecture, she met a man who was reflexologist that did work in the client's home. She was convinced that she had attracted him because of her focused thoughts and efforts to do all she could to heal the cancer.

Louise realized that she needed to love herself more. She had learned that in her church. She had taught this same concept to her own clients, but now it was her turn to use the power of her own belief system and thought process to help in her healing process. Prior to her cancer diagnosis she had not applied these principles to herself, but now she permitted herself to say, "I love you, Louise." She found a good therapist and worked through her emotional baggage, slowly letting go of her resentment and anger over her past.

Louise explains that she found a good nutritionist who helped her to detoxify her body. Not only did she clear the junk food out of her system, but also her junk food thoughts. Louise moved herself into a positive realm, letting only positive thoughts enter her conscious mind, and returned to the doctor's office six months after her diagnosis. They tested her and found no trace of the cancer. She had healed herself!

In Louise Hay's case, she was able to heal herself with a change of her thought processes and her beliefs about herself. However, she did confer with doctors and with other alternatives. This is not to say that we can always heal ourselves and that doctors should not be seen or listened to. I'm using Louise Hay's story as an example of the impact of a healthy self-image and a belief that we can be healed and live healthier. Our mental outlook is a definite factor in our health and how quickly we recover from any medical procedure.

Louise went through months of intense counseling and mind and body work. She learned that what had started as something tragic could become a wonderful learning opportunity for her. Not only did she heal her cancer, but she also healed her spirit. The whole experience gave her a new and valuable way of looking at life, and the experience changed her priorities. She closed her practice in New York and took a train to California, and after a thirty-year absence from Los Angeles, she contacted her mother and estranged sister to rebuild those relationships again. Although her stepfather was dead, she was able to forgive, and her mental and spiritual healing continued.

Louise Hay took the opportunities for physical healing and for clearing old energy and misunderstandings through her writing. In 1988, her book, *Heal Your Body*, was being sold in 33 different countries and read in 25 languages. Drawing on everything she had learned and experienced, she brought a positive philosophy and healing techniques to the world. Louise Hay inspired me to inquire deeper into this field. I, too, want to help us learn how to create more of what we want and enjoy a healthier mind, body, and spirit.

Personal internal work and courage to act in spite of our fear and move through that fear begins internally and reveals itself externally. Louise L. Hay's teachings are about the connection between what we think or believe and how that illuminates itself in our mental and physical health. However, I want to warn readers that in no way am I telling anyone not to seek medical help. I believe that we need the expertise of physicians who are able to treat us for whatever our physical health concerns are, but we also cannot underestimate the power of our thoughts in relation to our healing. Sometimes it takes a combination of the medical field, metaphysics, and alternative healing methods to regain good health.

Louise L. Hay was able to cure her cancer through alternative methods and the metaphysics of her thought process. She didn't ignore the medical field; she took responsibility and researched everything that she could to heal her from cancer. I've experienced healing myself through the use of a positive thought process and belief system, and I have seen my patients do the same thing.

I perform mostly surgical procedures in my office. People have a desire to have a healthier smile, and they come to me for either periodontal surgical treatment or placement of dental implants. I have found it critical to interview my patients prior to providing them surgical care. I have found that if the patient doesn't truly and 100 percent believe that they will heal well from the procedure then I don't recommend proceeding. If I do the same procedure on two different individuals, I have literally witnessed the positive attitude patient, the one who believes in me and in their ability to heal, will heal with fewer complications and discomfort. On the other hand, the patient that immediately inquires about the failure rate, possible complications, and so on seems to attract those into his life as he imagines them. I totally believe what we think about we attract.

I also believe that each one of us can be healthier and happier if we have the insight and courage to go through a transformation from the inside. By reflecting on our thoughts and feelings, we can begin understanding physical transformations. Many times people with recurring or chronic conditions are suffering because they don't believe that they can get better. People who believe that they can heal or recover from an illness or condition are more likely to get better sooner.

The human body's ability to heal itself is incredible, and this is impacted by what goes on in our minds. It is critical to understand the link between the two. The mind directly impacts the vibration of the body. Consider our thoughts. Do we generally think of ourselves as healthy or unhealthy? Our thoughts affect our quality of life, as well as our emotional status. Ultimately, all of our results are affected by our thoughts.

With this philosophy as our foundation, as long as we choose to focus on positive thoughts, our health will be a reflection of our state of mind. Positive, optimistic people enjoy good health, satisfaction, and joy. Conversely, people who choose negative thoughts frequently suffer from more illness and complications from surgical procedures. Which will we choose?

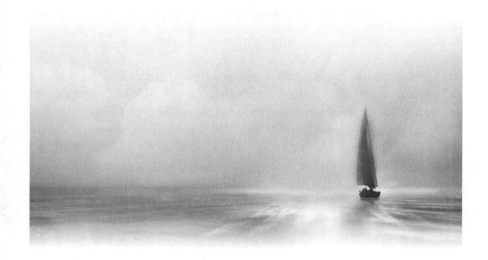

Chapter Six

—Forgiveness—

*When you hold resentment toward another, you are
bound to that person or condition by an emotional
link that is stronger than steel. Forgiveness is the only
way to dissolve that link and get free.*

—Catherine Ponder

Chapter Six

The subject of forgiveness may seem like an odd topic for a book about health, but these are strongly intertwined. A person's mental state has much to do with whether or not they become ill and if they recover well or develop chronic problems. When someone we care about hurts us, many of us will hold onto that anger, but this is not healthy. The building resentment and thoughts of anger put us into a very low negative vibration that attracts more of the same into our lives. Nearly everyone has been hurt by the actions or words of someone they trust or care about. Our sister criticizes our parenting skills, or a close friend reveals a confidence to another. With family, it can extend very deep in our hearts—consider the emotions we would experience if our spouse has been unfaithful or there is a past estrangement that has lasted for years. These hurts bring about stress and lower our resistance to disease. It is very common for an individual to have a falling out with someone close to them and find themselves quite unwell weeks, months, or even years down the road from the pent-up anxiety they have been carrying.

Time honored wisdom espouses that we should always forgive and forget, but that is easy to say and often hard to do. However, when we don't practice forgiveness, we may be the one who pays most dearly. By embracing forgiveness, we embrace peace, hope, gratitude, and joy, all of which raise our vibration levels and allow us to attract positive, healthy thoughts into our lives. The ability to forgive can be a lifesaving skill, as it will prevent years of anguish that may manifest as heart disease or cancer.

While there's no one definition of forgiveness, in broad terms, forgiveness is a conscious decision to let go of resentments and thoughts of anger toward another. Forgiveness is the act of releasing ourselves from thoughts and feelings that bind us to the perception that an offense was committed against us. This can reduce the power these feelings otherwise have over us so that we can a live healthier and happier life in the present. Forgiveness can even lead to feelings of understanding, empathy, and compassion for others.

One of the big misnomers about forgiveness is that to forgive somehow means we are condoning the actions of another person, which is not true. Forgiving does not mean that we have to enter into a relationship with that person. For example, if we were hurt or abused as a child, we can forgive the abuser but not have a relationship with them. The forgiveness is for our healing, not the other person's. If they ask for forgiveness and we can honor this request, that is more for their benefit. The forgiveness I am referring to, however, is our forgiving events in the past so we can heal and move forward without this negative energy in our heart, and this does not necessarily include reestablishing relatedness with that individual.

Forgiving doesn't necessarily mean forgetting either. The incident or event remains a part of our lives, and we decide how that impacts the rest of our lives. The wonderful thing about forgiveness is that it allows us to move on and stop focusing on the event. Forgiveness doesn't mean that we deny the other person's responsibility for hurting us, and it doesn't minimize or justify the wrong. We can forgive the person without excusing the act.

Researchers at Stanford University have been conducting ongoing research (known as the Stanford Forgiveness Project) looking into the long-term health effects of forgiveness. Evidence is mounting that demonstrates holding onto grudges and bitterness results in mild to severe health problems over time. Forgiveness, on the other hand, offers numerous benefits, including:

Lessening of anxiety symptoms

Decrease in chronic pain

Increased number of friendships

Healthier relationships

Greater spiritual well-being

Improved psychological well-being

Lower blood pressure

Stress reduction

Less hostility

Better anger management skills

Lower heart rate

Lower risk of alcohol or substance abuse

Fewer depression symptoms

Why do some people overcome past hurts and some don't? The reality is that this is a choice. Some people choose to move on and let the pain go, while others choose to keep the memory and pain. Much like picking at a scab, revisiting it mentally keeps the wound open and festering.

When we experience hurt or harm from someone's actions or words, whether this is intended or not, we may begin having negative feelings such as anger, confusion, or sadness, especially when the hurt came from someone close to us. These feelings may start out small. But if we don't deal with them quickly, they can grow bigger and more powerful. They may even crowd out positive feelings leading to both short-term and long-term health issues. Grudges filled with resentment, vengeance, and hostility take root when we dwell on hurtful events or situations, replaying them in our mind many times.

Soon, we may find ourselves entombed by our own bitterness or sense of injustice. We may feel trapped and not see a way out. It's very hard to let go of grudges at this point, and so instead we may remain resentful and unforgiving.

When we hold onto pain, old grudges, bitterness, and even hatred, many areas of our lives can suffer, including our health. When we're unforgiving, we pay the price over and over. We may bring our anger and bitterness into every relationship and new experience. Our lives may be so wrapped up in the wrong that happened in the past that we can't enjoy the present. Some signs that it may be time to let go and forgive include:

- Dwelling on the events surrounding the offense—and not just dwelling on them but remembering in them in glorious detail

- Receiving feedback from others that we have a chip on our shoulder or that we're wallowing in self-pity

- Being avoided by family and friends because they don't enjoy being around us

- Having angry outbursts at the smallest perceived slights

- Often feeling misunderstood

- Drinking excessively, smoking, or using drugs to cope with our pain

- Having symptoms of depression or anxiety

- Being consumed by a desire for revenge or punishment

- Automatically thinking the worst about people or situations

- Regretting the loss of a valued relationship

- Feeling like our lives lack meaning or purpose

If we insist on letting old hurts dominate our thoughts, we may often feel miserable in our current lives, and this adversely affects our health and well-being.

Forgiveness is a commitment to a process of change. It can be difficult, and it can take time. Everyone moves toward forgiveness a little differently. One step is to recognize the value of forgiveness and its importance in our lives at a given time and to our long-term health. Another is to reflect on the facts of the situation, how we've reacted, and how this combination has affected our lives. Then, as we are ready, we can actively choose to forgive the one who has offended us. In this way, we move away from our role as a victim and release the control and power the offending person and situation had in our lives. Forgiveness also means that we change old patterns of beliefs and actions that are driven by our bitterness. As we let go of grudges, we'll no longer define our lives by how we've been hurt, and we may even find compassion and understanding.

Forgiveness can be very challenging, especially with family. It may be particularly hard to forgive someone who doesn't admit wrong or doesn't seem to show remorse. Keep in mind that the key benefits of forgiveness are for us. If we find ourselves stuck, it may be helpful to take some time to talk with a person we've found to be wise and compassionate such as a spiritual leader, a mental health provider, or an unbiased family member or friend.

It may also be helpful to reflect on times we've hurt others and on those who have forgiven us. As we recall how we felt, it may help us to understand the position of the person who hurt us. In any case, if the intention to forgive is present, forgiveness will come in its time.

Please note that just because we forgive, it doesn't always mean reconciliation. In some cases, reconciliation may be impossible because the offender has died. In other cases, reconciliation may not be appropriate, especially if we were attacked or assaulted. But even in those cases, forgiveness is still possible even if reconciliation isn't. On the other hand, if the hurtful event involved a family member or friend whose relationship we otherwise value, forgiveness may lead to reconciliation. This may not happen quickly, as we both may need time to re-establish trust. But in the end, our relationship may very well be one that is rich and fulfilling.

The issue of forgiveness frequently arises when one family member is chronically or terminally ill. All parties are thrown together with the understanding this could be the last chance to grasp the wonderful release of forgiveness. These situations are difficult. If the hurt involves a family member, it may not always be possible to avoid him or her entirely. We may be invited to the same family holiday gatherings, for instance. If we've reached a state of forgiveness, we may be able to enjoy these gatherings without bringing up the old hurts. If we haven't reached forgiveness, these gatherings may be tense and stressful for everyone, particularly if other family members have chosen sides in the conflict.

Forgiveness may result in sincerely spoken words such as "I forgive you" or tender actions that fit the relationship. But more than this, forgiveness brings a kind of peace that helps us go on with life and adds to our overall well-being. The offense is no longer front and center in our thoughts or feelings. Our hostility, resentment, and misery have made way for compassion, kindness, and peace. Also, remember that forgiveness often isn't a one-time thing. It begins with a decision, but because memories or another set of words or actions may trigger old feelings, we may need to recommit to forgiveness repeatedly.

We cannot focus on getting the other person to change their actions. Another person's behavior or words isn't the point of forgiveness. In fact, the other person may never change or apologize for the offense. Think of forgiveness more about how it can change **our** lives by bringing us more peace, happiness, and emotional healing. Forgiveness takes away the power the other person continues to wield in our lives. Through forgiveness, we choose to no longer define ourselves as victims. Forgiveness is done primarily for ourselves, and less so for the person who wronged us. Once this victim mentality is released, our vibration escalates, bringing a more positive outlook and understanding of life. All of this results in better health and vitality.

What if we are the ones who did something wrong? Part of this process is that we must learn to forgive ourselves as well. It may help to spend some time thinking about what we have done and trying to determine the effect it has had on others. Unless it may cause more harm or distress, consider admitting the wrong we've done to those we've harmed, speaking of our sincere sorrow or regret, and specifically asking for forgiveness—without making excuses. However, if this seems unwise because it may further harm or distress those we care about, don't do it. Making ourselves feel better by apologizing is a selfish act unless it actually helps the situation. We don't want to reopen a painful wound. Also, keep in mind that we can't force someone to forgive us. They will need to move to forgiveness in their own time. In any case, we have to be willing to forgive ourselves. None of us is perfect, nor will we ever be. Holding onto guilt or resentment against ourselves can be just as toxic to our health as holding onto resentment against someone else. Recognize that poor behavior or mistakes don't make us bad—what happened is just what happened. When we release the guilty feelings from our minds, it allows room for the healthy, healing thoughts.

There are many physicians who actually have written about the association between cancer and suppression. Suppression here means keeping emotions bottled up and suppressed in our minds. A leading psychiatrist has said that most cases of mental disorder of the functional type are due to a sense of guilt. Many of us have grown up with guilt from our past. These emotions become a very powerful force in our subconscious minds and can really affect our physical health as well as our emotional health. I think Maxwell Maltz put it very well in his book, *Psycho Cybernetics*. He said that guilt is never an appropriate emotion.

We must accept ourselves despite our faults and admit our mistakes. Commit to treating others with compassion, empathy, and respect. And again, talking with a mentor, mental health provider, or trusted friend or relative may be helpful. Forgiveness of ourselves or someone else, though not easy, can transform our lives. Instead of dwelling on the injustice and revenge, instead of being angry and bitter, we can move toward a life of compassion, mercy, joy, kindness and peace. It takes a big person to forgive, but once we release this negative energy from our hearts and minds, we are free to allow more peaceful, healing energy in as we walk on our journey toward inner healing.

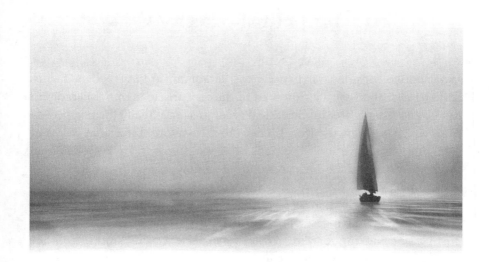

Chapter Seven

—New Paradigms and Habits—

*First we form habits, then they form us. Conquer
your bad habits, or they'll eventually conquer you.*

—Dr. Rob Gilbert

Chapter Seven

What do we consider our paradigms? Paradigms are our beliefs, habits, and feelings, and they all are stored in the subconscious mind. Paradigms can be and usually are self-limiting. Paradigms are actually the perspective from which we view the world. They are the way we think. In a way they form the glasses we look through as we see the world we spoke about in Chapter 1. So if we believe we are generally unhealthy, then we will generally be unhealthy, and not only will our health suffer, but it will be difficult for us to climb away from that paradigm. But it can be done. Our paradigm has to change from a mind-set that is negative to one that is positive and looking forward. When we experience this kind of conflict, we need to tap into our power to choose the thoughts we allow to enter our conscious mind. This can happen through our five senses, but more importantly it happens through our higher power intellectual faculties.

Our lives right now are the sum of the choices that we have made. We can choose all the thoughts that enter our mind, but if we really want to achieve our goals, then we need to be willing to make the choices necessary for achieving them. Also, we need to decide what we are willing to give up to achieve these goals. Now I don't mean we have to surrender our lives. We don't have to give up the things we love, but we do have to give up some old thoughts, habits, and beliefs. Many people give up their dream to travel the world because they hold a paradigm or a way of thinking that has them believing it's dangerous or simply not responsible. That is a paradigm in itself (what is responsible anyway?). We didn't talk to that attractive person because our paradigm has us believe we aren't good enough. We don't have to succumb to this feeling, but in order to dream we need to let go of the past, the old beliefs, the old self image, and old paradigms. We need to consciously choose actions and thoughts that will bring us closer to our goal.

A friend of mine named Susan has a daughter who recently graduated from college. Susan told me that her daughter was unhappy with her life. She said her daughter started to realize that things were becoming more and more out of control. She said she first started noticing it when she completed college. This strange time period of graduating college, becoming financially independent, and looking for a job was exciting in the beginning. She loved it. The thrill of seeking out a good job, having money, finding a place to live in the funky part of town seemed like what she should be doing, but once she did all that she began to ask herself, is this it? Once she had reached her short-term goals she felt unfulfilled, and every day turned into a routine. As time passed, the daughter said, "Every night when I go to bed I think, what did I do today? What difference did I make in the world today?"

My friend's daughter was used to her college paradigm of goal, reward, new goal, reward, another goal, reward. But these were small goals that were obtained and achieved quickly. She'd study and then she'd receive the A. She was used to instant gratification. If she was going to be happy, she was going to have to change her paradigm and see her life as a long-term endeavor with long-term goals.

Helen Keller said that when one door closes another one opens. All too often people are concentrating on the closed door and don't even notice the open door. Using visualization and repetition, we will develop the ability to see the door of opportunity immediately when it opens in front of us. Napoleon Hill said in his book *Think and Grow Rich*, "If we practice these principles long enough then riches will come to us so fast that we won't even know where they are coming from." He is referring to riches in *all* aspects of our lives, not just money.

Remember, our results are directly caused by the image we hold of ourselves, so if we change the picture we have in our subconscious minds and get rid of these limiting beliefs, we can change the results.

I remember when I was a child I was always told by my father that I had talent in science and math. I was not encouraged to take the top classes in English or literature. My self-image was that I was not a good writer. When I started thinking of sharing my ideas by writing a book, I really thought that I couldn't ever do that. I was letting my past (which created my paradigm) influence my future possibilities. But once I understood that this paradigm wasn't true, I started using these principles. I realized that, in fact, I can write a book. I found my open door, which was working with a publishing company that helps me through all the steps. I changed the way I looked at myself and the dream of writing a book is now a reality.

How do we change the paradigms? Remember, we were given the ability to think, and now we know how to choose what goes into our conscious minds, and therefore we can influence our subconscious minds where the paradigms are held. By becoming emotionally involved with our new thoughts, we will cause new actions, which then affect our results. The image we impress upon our subconscious minds controls our vibrations, and our vibrations controls all we attract into our lives.

Repetition

Repetition is one of the most beautiful things in the world. Think about anything we understand to be attractive or appealing. Art, music, design, dance, all have repetition at their foundation to make them wonderful. A song uses repetition in rhyming to make sense and to let us sing along. A painting uses repetition to complete the painting and to balance it out. And if repetition can bring beauty to these things, imagine the beauty it can bring to our lives.

Repetition is one of the keys to changing our paradigm. It is the first law of learning. The number of times we are exposed to something is really what makes the difference. For example, if we read the material presented in this book just 15 minutes every day, we will not only learn the material but we will develop a habit. The concepts, information, and action steps will be so ingrained in our minds we couldn't break it even if we tried. If we study something for just 15 minutes every day, at the end of a year we will have almost 100 hours of study! Small changes every day add up to a very big change in our results.

Repetition helps everything in the world make sense. It brings clarity, emphasis, amplification, and emotion to something that otherwise has none. A runner is not necessarily impressive if they jog a mile, but the repetition of miles until that distance becomes a marathon suddenly becomes awesome! Repetition inspires awe. Think about "Hey Jude," the last song on *Let It Be*, by the Beatles. That chord progression by itself, played one or two times through, has a nice sound, but that's it. But repeat that progression for several minutes and it takes on a certain power. Those chords, simply through the use of repetition, become hypnotic.

There's incredible power in repetition. If repetition can make millions of people weep when they hear a song, just think what repetition in our lives can do.

Visualization

Remember that great line in the movie *Field of Dreams*, "If we build it, they will come"? Visualizing something unimaginable can be magical. Now of course, building a baseball field in an Iowa cornfield may not make old baseball legends appear, but visualizing a new self image, a new paradigm, can create a new life.

Visualization helps the way we see the world. Think of our visualization as something we create. We see it in our mind, and therefore we have already begun to take the steps necessary to achieve it. If we know what it looks like in our mind, then it becomes real and tangible. This is actually how the Law of Attraction works once we are crystal clear on what we want. We will become more aware of the opportunities and situations that bring us closer to our goal. Then we just have to act on them.

Think of a blueprint used by an architect. Before that blueprint was laid down, that person visualized what they wanted to happen. They created power by visualizing their design and attracted the events to happen. When we visualize a goal, we alter the environment around us. We see in our imaginations what we want, and by keeping this vision fresh, by keeping this goal in our hearts (subconscious minds), our goal will inevitably come to us. Visualization combined with repetition causes our subconscious minds to hold our goal as true, and it is only a matter of time before this goal will be realized in our lives.

I had a patient named Russell, and he required a certain surgical procedure done. It was relatively costly, and from what I could tell, Russell was not interested in investing in his oral health. I was somewhat reluctant to tell him the news, but I realized that by letting these negative thoughts enter my mind, I was putting myself in a negative vibration, and I was setting myself up for a very bad encounter.

So I visualized myself greeting this man calmly and comfortably. I visualized Russell walking through the door with a smile on his face, the sun coming in behind him. I saw myself greeting Russell warmly, and him returning this graciousness with cooperation and friendliness. Then I visualized myself telling him about the surgery. I was grateful that I could help his situation and it really could help him reduce the infection he was experiencing and restore his oral health. I visualized him smiling and agreeing. I repeated this event over and over until it became part of my subconscious mind.

Through my visualization and repetition, I soon felt like the conversation had already happened, that Russell already agreed to have the treatment, and was grateful to move forward. Not surprisingly, when he walked in, Russell was smiling and friendly and completely agreed with the procedure. In the end, he did amazingly well through it all. Thoughts are the seeds to success so, when we nurture them with positive vibration and let them grow, amazing changes will result in our lives.

The Universal Laws

We live in a world and a universe that is organized and functions under seven universal laws. Each is an active part of nature and is as old as the universe itself. When we work in harmony with the universal laws, our lives and health take on a natural and easier flow. The seven universal laws are the Law of Vibration and Attraction, the Law of Gender, the Law of Cause and Effect, the Law of Polarity, the Law of Perpetual Transmutation, the Law of Relativity, and the Law of Rhythm. These natural laws apply to our solar system, our planet, and to us personally. They affect each one of us whether we are aware of them or not. They are at work daily, just like gravity.

We can live healthier and more physically fit lives by tapping into all the tools available to us. We have learned the basics about awareness and using our intellectual faculties; we changed our self-image and changed our attitude to one that reflects what we truly want in life. These thoughts are going to be at work whether we use them or not. I believe it is better to use them as tools in helping to create a healthy, prosperous, and successful life.

The Law of Vibration and Attraction

In his famous book, *Working with the Law*, Raymond Holliwell begins his chapter on the Law of Attraction with: "To desire is to expect, to expect is to achieve." These two very important phases of the law represent the mental attitudes of the attractive force. He goes on to explain that desire without expectation is idle wishing or dreaming. Desire literally helps to raise your level of awareness for the thing you desire, to connect you emotionally with it, and then expectation is like the gravity pull drawing you toward it.

Everything in the universe vibrates. Mind is movement, and the Law of Vibration states that everything moves constantly; nothing rests. Rhonda Byrne highlighted and created amazing publicity about the Law of Attraction in her movie, *The Secret*, but this law has also been written about by many other authors. The Law of Attraction conveys the idea that we are always moving toward something, and it is always moving toward us. This is also where our intuitive factor is used to pick up other people's vibrations. (A vibration can also be described as our feelings, once we become consciously aware of them. We might say "I feel bad, sad, or great," but what we are really declaring is that we are aware that we are in a negative or positive vibration.) So we are constantly sending off our feelings and thoughts into the universe through our vibrations. Our thoughts dictate our vibrations, so by changing our thoughts we can literally change the energy we are sending out into the universe! People around us can pick up these vibrations. Have you ever walked into a room of strangers and instantly had an opinion about the people? We might say that we could sense something in the room. These are the vibrations of the people that we are picking up.

A simple explanation for the Law of Attraction with regard to our health is that when we think, whether the thought is good, bad, or indifferent, we bring that circumstance into our lives. If we are focusing on achieving good health and fitness, then we are attracting those aspects into our lives. We may not actually realize that we are desiring a certain level of health and fitness, but based on our paradigms and beliefs, we do often expect to either be healthy or not.

If you have been diagnosed with cancer and the doctor says, "With the proper medicine and a good attitude you can beat this," she is not being flippant or offering a panacea. She is helping you to keep hope and thus maintain a positive attitude. This is critical, and it is a key point of this book. The Law of Attraction works like a magnet. Moving ourselves into a positive vibration will, without a doubt, increase our chances of overcoming a disease.

In the universe everything vibrates—nothing rests. Even down to the smallest atom, particles are constantly moving. Our conscious awareness of vibration is called "feeling." Our thoughts control our vibration and thus control our emotions. When we aren't feeling well, it is because we have sent out that vibration and have attracted something negative into our lives. This vibration is how the Law of Attraction works, and when we learn to choose positive thoughts we can alter our vibrations or feelings into positive emotions.

By moving into a positive vibration we will find that we are attracting the things we need to be healthy. It is really all about increasing our awareness of these things. Changing our eating habits to healthier food may be complemented when we learn about a new restaurant that just opened up in our neighborhood that serves organic foods grown locally. A new staff member at the gym where we work out each week has just arrived and his specialty is the exact help we need. We have heightened awareness of these things, so when they become available we are more likely to take action on them. We are attracting what we need to us, and they are a confirmation of our thoughts.

The circumstances and conditions of our health now are a result from our past attitudes, i.e., thoughts, feelings, and actions. By changing our attitude in a positive direction that focuses on what we want in our lives and with our health, the Law of Vibration and Attraction must bring the equivalent back to us. It's like picking up a television signal from a satellite. Our bodies and our minds work just the same. If we learn to change our attitudes toward our health, and therefore, change our desires and expectations of it as well, we will find ourselves attracting an entirely new and healthier existence.

The Law of Gender

Every seed has a gestation period. A plant takes time to grow, time to produce a fruit. When a farmer plants a seed, he knows how long it will be before the plant emerges from the soil. The gestation time is known. Our thoughts and ideas have a gestation period as well, except this time is unknown to us. The Law of Gender says that thoughts and ideas are spiritual seeds and take time to grow and manifest themselves into our physical reality. We tend to want to rush things, and we get frustrated when they don't manifest immediately. When we set our goals, they will manifest when the time is right, so we must be prepared for them to take time.

According to the Law of Gender, there is a right time for everything. So often we attempt to force or push because we are impatient to see the results we want in an unrealistic time frame. Once you understand this law, I hope that you will know that while we cannot control the time, we must continue to hold our goals in our hearts. Since there is a right time for everything, we need to be patient and believe that the goal we are focusing on will happen at just the right time for us. Too often people get excited and say they are going to change their lives, and they want immediate results. No one wants to wait or be patient. Unfortunately, some people only spend a short time focused on the goal, and they lose interest or give in to doubts and go back to their old habits before they can manifest their desire.

It is important for people to know that the Law of Gender works; it just *is*. We need to realize that if one thing does not work out for us when we want it to, something else will come along, and it may be even better than we imagined. When it comes to the Law of Gender, patience and persistence are key for us to remember!

The Law of Cause and Effect

The Law of Cause and Effect is probably the most familiar to people. For every action, there is a reaction. Remember, there is no such thing as chance—like causes produce like results. Everything happens according to law. It is like dropping a pebble in the water. The pebble causes ripples to form, and they continue across the water until they hit the other side. In the same way, what we choose to do or not do has an effect on us, as well as others.

Think about this in terms of our health. Since we are interested in the results in our lives to change, we need to focus on cause and the effect will automatically occur. This is the law. If we create a healthy environment, if we think "I maintain a balanced diet and I exercise regularly; I'm healthy," then we are sending positive thoughts out into the universe. Therefore positive outcomes will come back to us, and our chances for retaining our health are much improved. Now this is not to say that if we continue to say we are healthy that we'll never be sick, but the chances decrease dramatically with this thought process. Don't forget—along with these thoughts, the Law of Attraction is also at work, so this individual is desiring and expecting health, and therefore this healthy individual is also usually living a healthy lifestyle, and therefore she experiences less illness and will have a speedy recovery from any surgery or illness.

This is the same for the people around us. Have you are ever witnessed someone who is angry? They are sending out angry, desperate, negative vibrations, and what kind of vibrations are they getting back from the people around them? These people wonder "Why me all the time?" I say, "You are the cause of your results," so when we look at what we are putting out to the world we can honestly evaluate why we get the results we see in our lives. We are the cause! The more anger we give out, the more anger we will get back in return. We can influence how people affect our own health. Happy, optimistic people attract happy, optimistic people, and they are almost always more healthy.

We have probably all experienced this law many, many times. We are aware that one thing causes another. We learned it as children by dropping things and crying until our moms or dads picked it up for us. We quickly learned that the actions we took got attention from our parents. If we wanted more attention, then we dropped the toy again. It sounds so simple when we explain it this way, but this is actually how simple this law is.

The Law of Polarity

The Law of Polarity is also familiar to most people and we have introduced it earlier in this book. It has been present all of our lives, but most of us have not thought about it as a law of nature. Basically, this law states that opposites exist everywhere, and these are equal and diametrically opposed. There would be no hot without cold; there would be no up without down. There are two sides to everything. A healthy side and unhealthy side. The Law of Polarity says that there is always an equal and opposite for every thought, feeling, or action. This can be a very powerful law for us to experience once we have put the law to work for us. This law brings to mind the intellectual faculty of perception. Think about it—for every situation or thought there is always another side of the situation, however difficult it is to see sometimes. For every bad thing in our lives there is a good, but sometimes it is deeply hidden and it is very difficult for us to see this side.

For example, when diagnosed with an illness, the Law of Polarity tells us that even if the doctors tell us a certain outcome is probable, there is also the possibility of an opposite outcome. For example, if the situation is a life-threatening illness, then it is also possible that we can live longer . Receiving the news that we have been diagnosed with a terminal disease is difficult, but at the same time we must know that we have a choice in what we do in our minds with this information, much like the story of Louise Hay and her cervical cancer. While I am not saying that terminal illnesses can be cured, I am suggesting that we at least have a choice in how we will live the remaining days on this earth: will we be negative and angry and thus attract more of the same, or will we be grateful for the days we have left and for the people who are providing care for us? If we realize that the Law of Polarity is at work, we will always have hope, and we will have the ability to view the situation from another angle—and that can make all the difference!

The Law of Perpetual Transmutation

The Law of Perpetual Transmutation states that energy is always moving and always changing into a physical form. The image we hold in our mind will materialize as results in our lives. We have the power to give energy to an illness or not. Have you ever been at work and everyone around you is getting sick, and then when you come down with an illness you say, "This doesn't surprise me at all," or "I knew this would happen"? We gave our energy to that worry. We gave our energy to that illness, and when put in those terms it seems outrageous, right? That's because it is. We can control where our energy goes. We control the power of elements around us. By giving our energy to healthy ideas we are actually taking a stand and fighting back against illness. What a completely empowering idea!

According to many scientists, including Einstein, energy is in constant change. It can move into physical form and back to pure energy again. We live in a world and universe going through constant change. Everything that we see or know is either growing or dying, increasing or decreasing. Think about when we look up at the night sky and see thousands of stars on a clear night. We could actually see millions if we had a strong enough telescope. I think the photographs that we continue to receive from the Hubble telescope are amazing and magnificent. One of the most interesting things to me about seeing these pictures is that the photographs we see now show what the stars looked like thousands or millions of years ago. The light of a star we see tonight actually might not even be there anymore. Nothing stays the same.

The Law of Perpetual Transmutation can also be applied to visualization and images in our mind. It is at work when we project our thoughts out into the universe. This law materializes our thoughts into our reality. It comes down to knowing that whatever energy we give out, we will get back in return. The natural laws work together, and some of them overlap with others.

It's important for us to maintain awareness and learn to consciously send out thought waves that are in harmony with what we really want. Our thoughts, feelings, and actions need to be in sync to maintain harmony with our desires. Make an effort to always choose the image that best portrays your true desires. Remember, the thoughts you focus on will expand, so be careful what you wish for!!

The Law of Relativity

This law states that all things are relative. Everything gets a value based on a comparison to something else. There is no big unless we define what is small, and the same can be said for fast and slow and so many others. We can look at our medical diagnoses using this law by comparing our diagnosis to possibly something less serious. Let's say we have been diagnosed with high blood pressure. Yes, this can be a precursor for a number of diseases, but it is also very manageable. We might have to change our diet, exercise more, reduce stress, and so on and so on, but in comparison to terminal cancer or massive heart attack, suddenly high pressure doesn't look too bad. The Law of Relativity puts things in perspective. If something unfavorable (a speeding ticket) is compared to something awful (an automobile fatality), the unfavorable event really doesn't seem that bad. Nothing is good or bad unless we relate it to something.

This is especially important as it relates to health. Let's say we become depressed. Depressed thoughts become negative thoughts and negative feelings, which will cause us to be in a negative vibration. Then, the more negative feelings we experience, the more negative thoughts will enter our conscious mind, which ultimately results in us feeling sick, run down, and tired. Thus, this becomes the beginning of what can be a downward spiral.

Thoughts of feeling tired and lacking energy cannot be realized until they are compared with someone who might be energetic and full of life. Similarly, we cannot be sad without comparing this to someone else being happy. What I'm saying is that when we find ourselves in any unfavorable situation—in this case we'll say our health—look around and realize that compared to something else it is only as bad as we allow it to be. Practice relating our situation to something much worse and the situation will look much better. Remember, nothing is good or bad; only our thoughts make it so!

The Law of Rhythm

When the tide goes out, the tide will come back in. When a tree drops its leaves in the fall, it will bud again in the spring. It is the creation and destruction of worlds. It's the cliché of what goes around comes around. The Law of Rhythm is the natural cycle of everything, and when it is understood, this law can be extremely calming and very reassuring.

Once we understand this law as it relates to our health, this natural cycle of things occurring, then we can shape how our health comes back around to us. For example, remember back to the Law of Polarity, when everything around us is measured on its to and fro. We can control how that pendulum swings. This law suggests not to fight it if we are down. When we are in the ocean and get stuck in a riptide, we don't swim straight for shore, we don't fight it, we swim through it, and we might have to even float for a while to regain our strength. This is what needs to happen when we face unfortunate events with our health. Focus on whatever is good in the situation. Find something to be grateful for, and know that we can swim through it and calmer areas lie ahead. By doing this we can be assured that good times are to come.

One of my mentors, Jim Rohn, talks about the seasons of life. This reminds me of this law. He discusses the seasons of life as they relate to the seasons of the year. During winter we can be cold and miserable, or we can enjoy the beauty of the snow and know that the spring will be here soon. When we learn to roll with the tide and enjoy and be grateful for the space we are in each moment, we will find joy and happiness somewhere inside of every experience! I have learned over the years that focusing on negative results keeps that cycle repeating itself until we choose to move on. Knowing this can help us stay positive when we are going through challenges with our health. Sometimes we may feel that we are in the winter of our health, but in fact, it is a season of our lives that we must experience to prepare us for the spring, summer, and fall. Jim Rohn also reminds us that there is a season to sow and a season to reap, and you need to do both to achieve the harvest, but you can't do them at the same time!

Understanding that the Law of Rhythm is a natural part of life's process will help us keep moving forward. Go ahead and burn the bridge to our past and keep going. Knowing how to leverage this law helps us limit the impact of negative or difficult situations, and we can expect more good things in our future—we will attract them! When you are in a downswing, do not feel hopeless. Know that the swing will change and things will get better. When? Well, that is influenced by the Law of Gender! You see now how all these laws are at work together?

I met Beth through a doctor friend of mine. She had an attitude that was so negative that everything was dismal to her. Beth had basically quit believing there was anything good in the world.

My friend had known Beth for many years, and she had gone through her life saying how horrible everything was. She had a troubled childhood. Her parents were abusive, and they drank too much. Happiness did not exist for her, and in the spring of 2002 she was diagnosed with breast cancer. Although she wanted to be happy and she claimed she truly did want to live a better life and that she wanted the quickest road to recovery, Beth chose to keep letting negative thoughts enter her conscious mind. She was unaware of the power of these negative thoughts on her health. Remember, the Law of Attraction states that you must desire it *and* expect it. I don't believe Beth did either!

Beth was a very angry individual. In her hospital room nothing was right. If the lights were too bright she'd yell for the nurse to turn the lights off, and then when she couldn't live in this "utter darkness" she'd yell for the nurse to turn the lights back on. If the room was too hot, it was uncomfortable. If the room was too cold, it was "frigid." The food was "horrible." Beth complained about the way the doctors and nurses treated her. Everything was horrible for Beth. As much as my friend tried to explain to her that she controlled her own happiness, that she was letting in these negative feelings, Beth wouldn't listen. She didn't believe such a thing existed.

Beth said, "How can I control what some doctor does for me? How can I tell a nurse to leave the lights on without saying anything to her?" She didn't understand that her attitude about these things was influencing her health.

As her physical condition became worse with the cancer growing and spreading, she fell deeper and deeper into isolation and depression. Her health was failing fast, and she truly believed that she couldn't control it. She died the following fall with no family or friends by her side.

Beth was about as far away from a positive vibration as we can get, and it ultimately destroyed her. But did she stop to think about her situation? If she had understood the universal laws and how they are always working, she could have seen the positive aspects going on around her. For example, she could have said, "Wow, whenever I press this button the nurse comes in here to help me and to make me more comfortable." Or even, "I am grateful that I have a thumb to press this button that calls the nurse!" And, "Look how the doctors are using the best medicine in the world on me right now! How lucky I am to be in hospital like this!" Instead of having gratitude, Beth had anger.

The laws exist whether we want them to or not and are ever present in our daily lives. They are also intertwined in all we do. Each action we take, thought we think, or feeling we have is a factor in what we create for our future. We are totally and completely responsible for our lives, and while that may seem overwhelming to some, it is a wonderfully empowering idea. Rather than just letting life wash over us in an endless wave of happenstance, we can take charge of our future and design the lives we want to live by understanding and using these laws to their greatest potential.

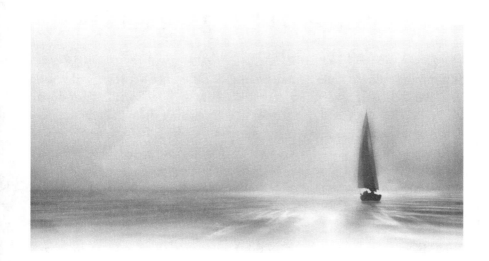

Chapter Eight

—Goal Setting and Goal Achieving—

A goal is a dream with a deadline.

—Napoleon Hill

Chapter Eight

It is important for people to understand the difference between goal setting and goal achieving. Very few people actually set goals, write them down, and follow up with action plans for accomplishing them. Therefore, very few people actually achieve them, and that is why success is a mystery to so many people. A goal doesn't have to be something huge. A goal can be little, like walking around the block. Small goals put together turn into big goals. Succeeding in that goal of walking more, combined with a goal of eating less junk food, can be the tools we need to achieve a bigger goal of losing five pounds.

I felt the same way about writing this book. Writing a book, when looked at as a whole, is incredibly daunting. I told this to one of my children, and she said, "Yeah, but Mom, if you write a chapter here and a chapter there, soon you'll have a few chapters. Put them together over a little bit of time and you've got a book." Her logic was breathtaking and totally inspiring. I used the faculty of imagination while working on this book. I imagined walking into my favorite book store and seeing it already published and on shelves. Throughout the process of writing and publishing I continued to really impress this goal into my subconscious mind. I imagined the excitement of seeing my book on the Barnes and Noble shelf in my local area. I have imagined the press release in national magazines. Local author writes book: *Mind and Medicine: In Harmony for Healing*!

I believe that one of the best tools to help us with our visualization is using a vision board. This is a poster board that holds pictures of all our goals and dreams so we can literally see it every day. This process may sound simple, but it is actually very profound and can help us become emotionally attached to our goal. Ultimately, through the Law of Attraction, these things almost miraculously will show up for us in our lives. An example of this for me is my boat. I had made a vision board about two years ago. I put a picture of a blue boat on it. At the time, I was married and we had a white boat and it was smaller than the boat in the picture. My husband at the time said to me, "Why do you have that picture of that big blue boat on your vision board when our boat is white?"

I had no idea that a few months after that conversation, I would find myself divorced and without a boat. At first, I figured that I could never achieve this goal of having my own boat. I found myself thinking that the beautiful blue boat would never be mine. In fact, I almost took those pictures off the vision board because I almost allowed the situation to steal my dream. Then I reasoned that I wasn't going to give into negative feelings. I was not going to become a victim of doubt and excuses and I kept the pictures up on the board and continued to hold the dream as possible. I desired it, expected it, and sure enough, an opportunity soon arose that allowed me to buy that beautiful big blue sailboat. Now, I am the proud owner of the sailboat *Harmony*.

What is your dream? Can you picture it in your mind right now? If we hold a picture of what we really want, then it is only a matter of time until we achieve it. We may not know when this will occur because we always have the Law of Gender at work. Remember, this natural universal law says that every idea, thought, or goal has a certain gestation period, and although we should put a time period onto our goal, we can't be attached to the time. We really don't know the time. We should get emotionally attached only to the outcome. We are working toward the goal, and it will show up for us when the time is right. We can change the time frame, but never change our goal. As Winston Churchill said: "Never, never, never give up!"

Why don't most people set and achieve big goals? I am going to suggest that this is due to the universal reason—fear. In Chapter 4, we discussed the terror barrier and how it affects our health as well as other areas. I know that I felt very fearful of owning my own boat. I was afraid I wouldn't be able to dock it and everyone on the dock would be watching me. This fear literally almost caused me to let go of my goal of owning my boat.

But again, from studying this material, I know that this was just a fear and didn't have anything to do with my potential. Now, I have my new boat, and I have learned to dock it very well. I did it while still afraid and overcame my fear, and I have achieved my goal. Goal achievers still have fear, but they just do it afraid and move through their fear and the terror barrier, and that is why they are successful.

When setting goals, remember there are two types of goals: logical goals and emotional goals.

Logical Goals

This type of goal is reasonable, and we do these for intellectual reasons. These goals make sense to us and are based on past results. They are safe. I have heard it said that if we are in sales and we have logical goals, we are going to have skinny kids. Confucius said, "Man who shoots at nothing is sure to get it."

Emotional Goals

These types of goals make us feel great when we accomplish them. These goals are much more powerful than logical goals. We don't want the boat, car, or house just to have them; we want them for the way these things make us feel. Our goals should excite and scare us at the same time. If it doesn't scare us, then it isn't big enough. Don't worry about how to get it. The steps to take will all be worked out in the process. I believe that no one knows how to accomplish a goal until they have completed it.

I like what Earl Nightingale said about success: it is the *progressive realization of a worthy ideal*. As long as our goal is worthy and we want it with all our heart and soul—and we are working toward it, then we are already successful. It is progressive so we are successful already, right now!

Stop and think a moment. What do you really want? I am suggesting that with this method you can think, dream, and fantasize past what your present results are. When you believe in yourselves and your abilities, you will be able to accomplish goals that may be over and above what you think you can do. It begins with thinking about what you really want—I encourage you to dream about it and focus on it.

If you have health issues, then set a goal for how you want to feel. Your thoughts and focus will help you to succeed in being healthier. Some of us may be in a situation right now that requires a medical procedure or surgery of some kind. Part of healing quickly and successfully is how we see ourselves now and afterwards. We can use an index card to write down how we want to feel and what we want to do after recovery. Write it in the present tense, as if it has already occurred. I use the format: "I am so happy and grateful now that …" We must see ourselves enjoying life again and having a smooth and short recovery. Whether your goal is for health and fitness or another aspect of your life, I encourage you to use your imagination and visualize what you want your results to be. Believe it and do it.

For most of us the hardest part is getting started. Don't wait until a better time. There is never a better time than now. Start right now and we are 50 percent done. There is an ancient Chinese proverb that says: " The longest journey begins with the first single step." We must make the decision to change our lives and our results. Know where we are going—where we want to end up. I promise we will each get there. The first step is our decision to do so.

> *If a person will advance confidently in the*
> *direction of their dream and endeavor to live the*
> *life they imagined, they will meet with success in*
> *uncommon hours.*
>
> **—Henry David Thoreau**

We might experience obstacles that keep us from achieving our goals. What thoughts or things could you remove from your life that would bring you closer to your goal? This could be to avoid listening to the negative media on your way to work, or possibly you need to change that habit of spending time with certain people who don't value health as much as you do. Do you need to avoid talking with individuals that get you down so you can maintain your positive attitude? Well, whatever that thing is for you, do it now. Make a decision and do it. I also recommend that you find someone to hold you accountable to it as well. I always find it encouraging and helpful to have an accountability partner that I can talk to every week. It helps keep me on track.

I know a woman, Deborah, who struggled with her weight for years. She was obese as a child and through the years, as she had children and aged, she gained even more weight. It wasn't until Deborah's doctor told her that she had early onset diabetes that she truly grasped the reality that this extra weight could seriously shorten her life. Though she'd been on diets before, every time it got difficult she reverted back to her old habits. Deep inside her subconscious mind Deborah held the paradigm that she couldn't lose the weight—that she was destined to live out her life as an obese person. As a child she'd been told repeatedly that her family was just large and so she would be as well. This paradigm lodged in her subconscious mind and was very strong.

Deborah used visualization to see herself as she truly wanted to be—healthy, fit, and one hundred pounds lighter. It was a staggering goal, but she set smaller, progressive goals and focused on the outcome, not on the struggle to get there. It took almost two years, but Deborah lost the weight and has kept it off. She will be the first to tell us that it wasn't about diet or exercise. It was about understanding how her mind worked and that she could change those ideas that were set into her subconscious so many years ago. Once those ideas were challenged, then her goals were able to manifest themselves in her life as reality.

Imagine your goal already accomplished, visualize it, become completely emotionally attached to the goal, and watch the results soar!

Bridge the gap between where you are now and where you truly want to be. Goal achievers have consciously or unconsciously made a decision—a decision I sincerely hope you will make here and now; be a goal achiever. Choose to be healthy and happy, set new goals, and go for them with all your heart!

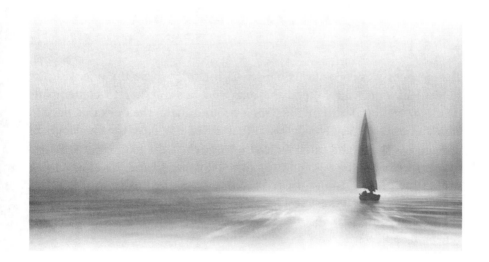

Chapter Nine

—Family and Loved Ones—

You are today where your thoughts have brought you; you will be tomorrow where your thoughts take you.

—James Allen

Chapter Nine

I sometimes wonder what is harder. Is it harder to be the one with the illness, the one who suffers, the one who possibly has to contemplate death; or is it harder to be the people around them, the ones that have to stand around seemingly helpless as their loved one faces the challenges of a diagnosis that could possibly lead to death? It's the one with the illness who is faced with the possibility of leaving this world and their loved ones, but it's the people around them, the loved ones, the husbands, the wives, the children, the mothers and fathers and brothers and sisters—those are the people being left. So what is harder, to be the one who leaves or the one being left?

The family is the most important life support system a patient can have. They are the ones who maintain happiness, instill confidence, and promote recovery. And because of this, they need to focus on several different things throughout the illness and the recovery process: hope, gratitude, positive energy, and thoughts. We all know the meaning of these words, what they symbolize. We know them so well that they almost seem generic and contrived, but what do they do when put in relation to well-being and health?

It is critical to have *hope*. We know the general idea, but for patients and families, hope is the difference between living and dying. The definition itself is related to better health: belief in a positive outcome related to events or circumstances in one's life. This perfectly embodies what we are trying to accomplish. By having hope in one's everyday life and in one's outlook, hope, for even the most difficult of all situations, is inevitable. This type of outlook must be maintained throughout any diagnosis, both by the patient and the family. If we think back to Chapter 6, when I described the seven laws, we will remember that to keep and maintain a positive mind-set, we must overwhelm ourselves with positive feelings and remember that our situation in life is subjective and controlled by us. But what about the family? Although we can't directly influence the patient's attitude, our attitude is definitely picked up by the patient and can directly influence the healing process. The family and friends too must understand the ideology behind the universal laws, because the families' hope is part of the patient's success.

Gratitude can be expressed in many ways. We buy flowers for our loved one. We listen to an elder tell their stories. Gratitude is an important part of attracting happiness into our lives. We talked about the vibrations of the universe and how we can move ourselves into those positive and negative vibrations. Gratitude, when felt in a truly sincere manner, is the highest level of attraction and vibration that we can have. For example, when we are looking at all the good in our lives, or seeing how much better off we are than something else, then our power of attracting more powerful positive vibrations is greatly enhanced. Yet, this process can sometimes be extremely difficult.

If we are ill it is easy to look around and not feel like we can find anything to be thankful for. How can someone be in a state of gratitude when everything around them is going wrong? It is important to recognize we are responsible for everything that is going on in our lives. We can't blame someone else for an illness. We must accept the fact that if, heaven forbid, something unfortunate does happen in our lives, we are the only ones who have any power over it, because remember, we become what we think about!

The universal laws are manifestations based on previous emotions. What we thought about and felt yesterday produces the results we see today. What we think about and feel today will produce results for tomorrow. We are the ones who originate our thoughts, so while we may want to blame someone else, the truth is that it is our responsibility. This maybe seems a bit harsh, but what a great feeling to know that we can, today, this minute, right now, change everything that will happen to us by changing or altering what we are thinking. Since we created the thoughts that led to our past results, isn't it reasonable to say that we can change our results by changing our thoughts, which will then change our emotions? So instead of seeing a diagnosis of our family member as a something we can't control, I am suggesting to express gratitude to those around us, let that carry over to our loved one and see how their health is positively affected. Be thankful for the time we have or have had. Although there is always something to be grateful for, I do realize however, this is not always easy to see.

Remember, nothing is good or bad; only our thoughts make it so. It is our perception of a diagnosis that makes it good or bad. A misguided perception, one that condemns a patient, can be based on false beliefs and insufficient knowledge. For example, to someone who has no knowledge of penicillin, a strep throat could possibly be seen as a life-threatening disease because their knowledge, their understanding, and their perception does not know that the illness can be cured in a week and half by simply taking medicine. Now strep throat and cancer are quite different illnesses, but in this example the patient's and the family's perception of the illness is exactly the same because of their awareness level. Wrong perceptions can be responsible for situations showing up in our lives in the form of events, illnesses, diagnoses, and circumstances.

Thoughts are what make us happy and sad; they are what help us gain back our health or lose it again. For the patient, knowing how to understand and use positive thoughts throughout the healing process is as great and powerful as modern medicine and is vital to accomplishing our goal of living a fulfilling life.

I can't stress enough how important it is for patients to bring only positive thoughts into their conscious minds. It might seem silly to think of the call button for the nurse as a blessing, or the fact that we still have a thumb to press it, but on the contrary, it is the smallest things that allow us to take these wonderful feelings into our subconscious minds and ultimately affect our outcome.

Family and Close Friends

But what if you're not sick? What if you're not the one who has the medical condition or, the one just diagnosed with an illness? The role the family plays in a successful recovery is huge because once one member of the family is diagnosed, that diagnosis impacts everyone.

So what can the family do? We, as family members, can greatly affect the way our loved one is feeling. We can bring about negativity—often times without even being aware of this energy, but this is extremely detrimental to the patient's recovery. We can do this by the looks and expressions we give, the things we say, the things we talk about. All of these send out a certain energy or vibration that is picked up by the patient, and studies clearly show that this can happen even if the patient is unconscious. To assist our loved ones recover, we must only be sending positive vibrations. And this must be done time and time again. Success for a patient relies heavily on our persistence.

Look at anything we have done in the past. Everything we have accomplished has been accomplished through persistence. An Olympic runner cannot become an Olympic runner without persistence. The president cannot become the president without persistence. Persistence is what intensifies the feelings in our lives. Now these feelings can be bad as well. Persistence is focusing the energy of one thought or action. It can be used to intensify a positive or negative thought or idea.

Persistence is a unique mental strength. It is a strength that is essential to fight against the seemingly overwhelming power of rejection, disaster, failure, and illness. We are all fighting something all the time. Persistence pulls us through by keeping us focused. It is generally believed that a lack of persistence is a consequence of weak willpower. This is completely untrue. In most cases, if a person lacks persistence, they do not have a goal worthy enough to keep them moving forward. For the family of a patient, persistence is critical.

I believe it would be the dream for the family and friends to see their loved one healthy and smiling again. I also believe this would be their number one goal. Persistence and positive thought are important in moving a person toward his or her goal. We are powered by desire and encouraged by the dreams we hold, and for the family and patient, that dream is health.

Here are a few things family members can focus on when dealing with an illness or condition in the family. Clearly defined goals are critical, and although we should think outside the box when making our goals, they cannot be unrealistic. For example, we don't set a goal of 100 percent health in one month for someone who has just been diagnosed with terminal cancer. Also, pick a goal that we will be emotionally involved in. I know this may sound ludicrous when dealing with illness in the family, because how could we not be emotionally involved with it? What I am suggesting is to set a goal such as, I will read a story to her every day, or I will eat my supper with her every night. Although, that goal may be relatively small, we will be emotionally involved, and these small goals lead to larger ones. Even if in the beginning we are a little doubtful of the final outcome, these small goals will plant the seeds in our subconscious minds and will allow the belief in the larger goal to follow.

Clearly establish a plan that the entire family can begin working on immediately. By setting down a plan, everyone knows what their roles are. This will give everyone a sense of worth throughout the process. Everyone is an integral part of the healing process. It is important to begin as soon as possible. Procrastination is detrimental to progress and positive thoughts. The longer we wait to take action, the more our mind will begin to doubt the situation, which will only foster negativity. Also, the sooner we get started, the more excitement and energy we will have. This energy will produce better results and more positive outcomes.

Make an irrevocable decision to reject any and all negative suggestions that come from an outside source, such as other family members, friends, neighbors, and coworkers. If someone's comment does not fit with your plan, then move along to the next idea or comment. Stay focused and persistent. Listening to negative influences can greatly alter the success of recovery, oftentimes resulting in the goal not being accomplished.

The difference positive energy from family members makes is amazing. Jennifer is my receptionist, and recently her dad suffered a tremendous injury when he fell from a ten-foot ladder onto the pavement. Jen's dad is fifty-seven years old and suffered four broken ribs, a fractured skull, three fractured vertebra, and a hematoma on the brain.

Jennifer worked hard with other family members to keep the energy in the room very positive and help her dad recover. Two days after the accident she says he woke up, meaning that he came to full awareness, even though he had been physically awake the entire time. Though his pain was excruciating at times, he never stopped thinking positively. He focused on the fact that he wanted to get back to work and support his family. He attributes the constant positive energy from his family as one of the main things that pulled him though.

He got out of the hospital into rehabilitation in record time, and Jen feels the attitude of the guests in the room was critical for his speedy recovery. This is not so obvious for a lot of people to understand because, especially in the beginning when her father was not very alert, it was very sad to see him, but it is important to always have a positive attitude around the patient. It is up to the family to support each other's sad emotions **outside** of the room so the patient doesn't pick up any of that negative energy **inside** the room.

My patient Rich shared his story in a letter he sent to me when he learned I was writing this book. He believes that his positive attitude directly affected his son's healing from a life-threatening condition.

On a bitterly cold and dark January night, a beautiful baby boy was born in a small Vermont town to the delight of his young and euphoric parents. Given that this was my first child, I anxiously watched and waited as the pediatrician carefully examined our newborn son from head to toe.

The doctor was all smiles as he concluded his positive report and only casually noted as he left the room that he had detected a mild heart murmur that should be of no concern given that 99 percent of these murmurs disappear within a few days of delivery. We couldn't have been happier. But that euphoria and happiness was to be short lived.

The following morning our son went into critical heart failure, and he was immediately moved into the small neonatal intensive care unit of our community hospital. Because of the rural nature of Vermont, the hospital did not have a pediatric cardiologist or the clinical capabilities to accurately diagnosis, much less, treat our newborn son.

After endless hours of waiting and worrying, we were finally informed that our son was born with life-threatening congenital heart defects that in all likelihood would prove fatal within the next few days. "We will make your son comfortable," the doctor said, "but there is nothing beyond that we can do for him given the seriousness of his condition."

Stubborn and impatient in the best of times, I adamantly refused to accept the doctor's declaration of defeat and immediately went into high gear, determined to save our young son's life. And thus began a 28-year journey that continues to this day.

We knew immediately that the most important thing we could do was to get our son to a hospital with the sophistication and medical staff equal to the medical challenges our son presented. We found such a facility at the Boston Children's Hospital, where it was soon determined that our son was born with over 30 holes in the septum between his left and right ventricles. We were told his chances of survival were less than 5 percent. This would not the last time we were given odds of this nature.

Over the course of the next 28 years, my son had over 12 open-heart and/ or pulmonary operations, a heart transplant in 1996, and a second heart transplant in 2006. And even during the darkest and most difficult hours, not once did I ever for a moment lose hope or confidence that we'd be taking our boy home for good. And never once did we ever feel pity for ourselves or our predicament. And that beautiful baby boy, who had only days to live, is now a fully functioning 28-year-old adult who stubbornly and impatiently refuses to let his illness bring him down. He lives every day knowing that hope, optimism, and science is the basis for every beat of his heart.

For the patient, let your family be a part of your recovery; and for the family, be there for your loved one. It's a hard and lonely thing to go through something like a serious or terminal illness without the support and love of people around us. For the family and close friends, remember that our energy, our vibration, will be picked up by the patient and will directly influence the thoughts, emotions, and ultimately the outcome of the patient.

My dad died of prostate cancer, but his words of gratitude were inspiring. Before he died he called me to his side and told me that the last few days had been some of the most special in his life. All of my siblings and his wife were gathered around him and stayed with him 24/7 for the few days prior to his passing. He saw how much we cared for him. But when he was telling me how much he loved us all and how much he appreciated everything that we'd done for him, the tears poured out and rolled down his cheek. We sang and prayed with him to keep the energy in the room as positive as it possibly could be.

Even as he was dying, my father was accepting positive feelings into his life. In his final hours he was smiling and sharing stories. The family was sitting at his bedside listening, enjoying, smiling, and even laughing. He kept the jokes coming until he could barely speak, and he kept us laughing even when we were very sad. Laughter is a wonderful thing, and we should remember to use it when possible. When he did close his eyes for the last time, we shed tears, of course, but we all understood that crying out of complete sadness would have been an injustice to this great man. We held each other and cried and smiled and felt his spirit with us. We were left with such an immense amount of uplifting emotions from him, and we couldn't help but feel joy from his life.

Joy can transcend death and the many trials of life. So I ask you to look for the good and offer gratitude. Be there for each other. Lift each other up when the other has fallen. Look at what you have in your life and smile about it, be thankful for it, find all the joy you can in it, fall in love with it, and then pass it on. Be persistent with it. And, finally, once and for all, share joy, laughter, and hope.

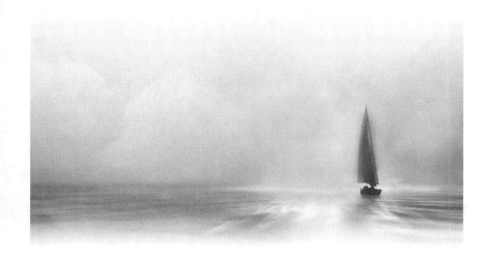

Chapter Ten

—For Physicians and Health-care Professionals—

It's no use saying, "We are doing our best." You have got to succeed in doing what is necessary.

—Winston Churchill

Chapter Ten

To be in health care, to be able to interact with and help patients, is a very privileged position. I cherish every moment I am able to spend with my patients talking to them, helping them with questions and concerns, and assisting them on their road to recovery. I consider my care to be very important in the overall health and well being of the patient. In our office, we don't fix teeth; we inspire and offer hope to our patients by making a difference in their lives through the treatment options and care we deliver for improved oral health. What I find to be challenging is explaining to my patients exactly what their diagnosis is (if their periodontal condition is very advanced) and what needs to happen during recovery from the surgical procedures I provide. This challenge is amplified when trying to emphasize the importance of positive thought processes for a patient who is afraid and feels lack of hope.

For the longest time, positive thinking and the universal laws were not endorsed by physicians. They brushed them off as nonfactual. If there is no scientific evidence, then how can it work, how can it be true? Physicians also thought that if there is no science backing it, then prescribing positive thinking to patients could be viewed as a scam or hoax not really helping their patients heal. But now, physicians have begun to change those antiquated ideas.

Researchers at Duke University have released details from a study conducted with patients who were diagnosed with heart disease for ten years. The patients were followed and asked about their mental states, their attitudes, and whether or not they were having negative or positive thoughts about their diagnosis. The study found that those patients who were feeling negatively about their chances of recovery at the time of the diagnosis were more likely to die within ten years than those who kept a positive outlook. This shocked the researchers. They were baffled. Finally we had definite evidence that positive attitudes are essential for health and recovery.

The researchers explained how they took various other factors into account as well, such as isolation, depression, and even the weather. Still, the positive-feeling patients battled the illness considerably better. Dr. Redford William, who is the director of the behavioral medicine research at Duke, claims that patients with a positive outlook and those who were able to put everything into perspective were 30 to 50 percent less likely to die during the ten-year period.

So for physicians and dentists who are wondering about positive thought, I am merely suggesting that we tell our patients that having a positive attitude will greatly influence their health for the better. We need to remember to tell them that having a positive outlook does not mean they should be blind to reality, but it is our duty to help them along, give them support, be their life coach throughout the recovery process. Through our encouragement, the patients will feel the comfort of having the support of a health-care professional advising them to see the world a bit brighter. People are smart when it comes to emotions, and we cannot hide them long term. If we simply smile and tell our patients that they need to think positively about their diagnosis, but we do not actually believe it ourselves, we will have the reverse effect of what we are trying to endorse.

We may be asking ourselves what we can do for our patients, how we can teach them how to live more positive lives when we aren't trained in the area of positive thought. Really, we are already aware of the path we have to take and lead them down. It is up to us to become confident in ourselves and what we say to our patients. They trust us. Most physicians know that after a diagnosis, even people with tremendous amounts of drive and determination have feelings of helplessness. We must help them—that is our obligation as health-care providers. We have to reassure them that they must maintain hope, and that they have the power to make that life-altering change in their recovery.

There will be many people in the medical field who will be looking to us as their support, and many of them will want to know the secret to good health. We can let them know that it is actually very simple, but few people realize this. Once we have increased our awareness of the impact of thoughts on our health, we can greatly influence the health of our patients. However, ultimately it is up to the patient to determine how they will view their diagnosis and respond to treatment.

Sadly, the majority of people never take the time to understand and develop how to take responsibility and change their attitude. People like being victims. They have been taught certain ideas throughout their lives—these thoughts are lodged deep in the subconscious mind—that counteract this new philosophy, but if they are willing to listen and make an effort to change their awareness level, they can learn how to change those old paradigms, change their attitude, and experience a new sense of freedom and health! Once patients realize that their thoughts can directly impact their outcome, then our job of coaching them will greatly change. We will no longer be the one to drive the recovery process. They will feel empowered by their own actions and will want to pursue their healthy mind/healthy body through more positive thoughts and feelings.

A huge percentage of people we come in contact with will believe the philosophy that accumulating more physical things will bring happiness and possibly even health. They will seek out such things as working more hours or buying more things, which scatters the mind, diffuses it, and makes it more susceptible to overwhelming emotions like exhaustion, depression, anxiety, and fear. This, of course, will only bring them more and more negative feelings. And because of this obsession with physical and material items, people knowingly and unknowingly overlook the unlimited supply of positive potential. It is easily within their grasp and yet they fail to grab at it. Remember the Law of Energy: nothing is destroyed or created. We have everything we need right here. We just need to develop a higher awareness level about it.

When we are sick, our illness seems to take over all of our thoughts. So if good health is one of the highest goals for most people, and obtaining it can occur often by changing our thoughts, then why wouldn't someone want to understand and implement this new way of thinking? The universal laws and principles are simplicity, safety, and comfort in the purest form. To teach our patients to become aware of and to develop an understanding of manifesting and consciously harmonizing their thoughts and feelings toward the positive can result in the difference between a life of joy, satisfaction, and good health or one of fear and anxiety; the latter, of course, will contribute to poor health.

Over the past twenty years, evidence has suggested that psychological factors can play a significant role in the development of coronary artery disease. It has been shown that positive thought provides encouragement for the body as it heals, so much that it has enhanced the effect of standard cardiac rehabilitation and reduced all-cause mortality and cardiac event recurrences for up to two years. This can happen just by thinking differently and releasing old negative thought patterns.

Both positive and negative emotions have a considerable influence on people's immunity and susceptibility to infection. After systematic exposure to a respiratory virus in the laboratory, individuals who had reported higher levels of stress and a negative attitude have been shown to develop a more severe and persistent illness than those who reported only positive emotions. The same results happened to individuals suffering various intensifications of the cold virus; those who maintained a positive emotional state were more associated with greater resistance than those who were in a negative state.

Those of us who are surgeons know the benefits of positive thought, and this is crucial before surgery. Pre-surgery is one of the most vital times to correct any doubt we or the patient might have. I know that I do visualization exercises in the morning prior to going into a surgical procedure. I prepare myself mentally by envisioning the surgery in my mind prior to actually lifting the scalpel to the patient. I envision the procedure being done successfully and without any complications. This is not unlike what I have read the Olympic athletes go through prior to performing their events. The visualization improves their performance in the events, and I believe it helps me in my surgical procedures as well.

A friend said that before surgery she had given a patient a CD with various steps on coping with stress and creating a positive emotional state. By doing so the patient was able to listen many weeks before the surgery, giving herself plenty of time to become familiar with this positive process. The CD consisted of guided imagery, calming music, and instructions to focus on only positive thoughts. She said that the patient who did this, who went through the CD and was able to do the activities on the CD, was able to recover more quickly from the surgery than other patients who hadn't listened to this CD or had done a similar kind relaxation exercise.

Similarly, I remember one time I was treating a patient named Yin. She was very young, and she was going through tremendously big procedures in which she was going to not only lose all her teeth, but she was going to need major bone reconstruction to redevelop the bone that was lost due to her periodontal disease. She was then going to have dental implants placed. She was very nervous, and she was asking me all kinds of questions as we were preparing for the first procedure. It would be the first of many large surgical procedures over the next few years. I remember sitting in my office talking with her about the importance of her state of mind on the outcome of the procedure. I told her that her state of mind and the attitude she brought to the surgery would have a direct effect on the outcome of the procedures. I told her that I too had to put myself in a positive mental state, and I shared with her that in fact, every day prior to going to work I journal and pray that my hands will be used as tools for God to heal my patients. I pray that my patients will trust me to work through a higher power to heal their bodies, but I also hope that they will allow my positive energy state to enter into their minds as they heal: body, mind, and spirit as one. I also told her about how I use visualization prior to surgical procedures and that I promised to do my part—that I would bring positive energy into the surgical room and that I really needed her to allow the energy to penetrate her mind and allow the healing to occur. I will never forget the faith that she obtained from that conversation. I could tell that she was going to really do well during the procedure, and her positive attitude was going to carry her through the difficult surgical procedures and through the entire healing time she would experience in the next few years until she had her healthy, happy smile back—but this time it would be with dental implants supporting it!

During the first procedure (and all subsequent ones), Yin brought in some relaxing music, and she literally was able to put her mind into a meditative state as I was doing the procedure. She chose not to have sedation, but explained that she could use the meditative music to relax her mind and receive my energy of healing. Of course I used plenty of local anesthesia, so she didn't feel anything, but the way she could alter her mind and allow the positive energy to flow through my hands of healing was one of the most memorable experiences of my entire career. It was her open mindedness and faith that allowed her to get through this life-altering situation with amazing success and surprisingly little pain or suffering. She believed in her mind, impressed this belief in her heart and so … it was!

Attitude can make a patient recover or fall deeper and deeper into the illness. Patients expect professionalism and encouragement from us as their health practitioners, and it is critical to realize how their optimism will reflect our attitudes. We cannot underestimate our attitudes to our patients healing and recovery.

In my own life I look toward joy, gratitude, and happiness as some of the most important aspects of life, because when we have joy in our hearts, everything else will fall into place. It is sometimes a challenge because many of the people in the dental and medical field these days are filled with a scarcity mind-set. Medical care providers are faced with an insurance crunch, which can greatly influence the care and support we can offer. I see many of my peers make choices for their patients and themselves based on scarcity, such as insurance and financial worries, as opposed to serving our patients, which is hopefully the real reason they entered the medical profession.

Therefore it is critical for both the patient and doctor to work from a place of gratitude, abundance, happiness, and ultimately freedom in their own lives. I heard it said that we will need 1.9 new doctors for every retiring doctor, because the new ones are working less hours and less days. This is largely due to declining compensation and personal satisfaction. I think it is important to address the health-care struggle and realize how it will impact our patients' care. I don't think the public at large has any sense that this crisis is approaching ever so rapidly.

I believe the doors of opportunity are in front of every health-care provider: to make a difference for our patients, to recommend and provide the best care for our patients, and to work toward more fair compensation for our services from insurance companies. I believe if we keep our focus on the care we provide and make choices based on our vision to serve our patients, then we will find both our financial needs and our patients' health needs fulfilled. Continue to find our door of opportunity and always remember, as Wayne Dyer said, "From abundance, we take abundance and still abundance remains." If we go to the ocean or to a wide-open beach and fill the biggest container we have with water or sand, there will still be an entire ocean or beach for us and the rest of humanity to draw from. But if we go to a place of less water or sand (where these resources are scarce), then we can fill up a container and deplete our source. We choose the source from which we live. Does it have walls of scarcity, or will we live and teach others from an abundant source? It is our choice. Learning to think in a new way is exciting for patients, but learning to assist our patients to heal in a new way is revolutionary for physicians.

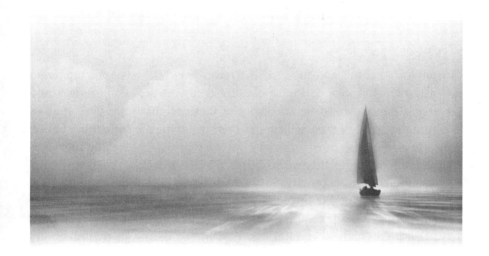

Chapter Eleven

—Hope—

Once we choose hope, anything's possible.

—Christopher Reeve

Chapter Eleven

Our ability to think and focus on whatever we choose is amazing. Even when the world looks dark and gloomy and wars are being fought and poverty is rampant, still we are a species that can choose to look at all of this in the world, see it as reality, and then still hope for something better. Hope is one of the most powerful forces that exist. Most of the good that has happened in this world has happened through hope. Anything worthwhile can be accomplished through hope. Alexander Graham Bell couldn't have invented the telephone if he wasn't hopeful it could be done. Martin Luther King Jr.'s speech of "I have a dream" wouldn't have been written if he didn't believe somewhere within us there was the possibility of hope. Hope is all around—we just have to tap into it.

Positive thinking is powerful and has unlimited potential. The results we can create when we embrace a positive attitude are infinite. When we use hope as our fuel the world opens up to us. For a moment, think about the different people in our lives: our family, our friends, coworkers, neighbors. When we listen to them, we start to understand just what makes them unique, the things they like, the things they have done. All of these are based on their hope for the future.

Positive thinking is often talked about in a flippant or trite manner. That couldn't be farther from the purpose of this book. I am using the term positive thinking as something we can learn to do with intention, so we can be the cause of our results. Positive thinking can be looked at as constructive thinking, and with constructive thinking comes gratitude. Gratitude is the cement for hope. It's the foundation. So why do people even talk negatively about things? As with many things that don't serve us, negative talk is easier. It is a habit. It is something we learn as children and are surrounded by in our adult life. It is part of our subconscious minds! It's often easier to focus on the negative in something than to search for the good. One could argue that it is a type of defense against things that go wrong and people who treat us poorly, but that is not necessarily true. Letting go of negativity can feel difficult in the beginning because we need to accept responsibility for our thoughts and actions, and most people do not want to do this. It is easier to blame someone or something and be a victim. If everyone around us is negative, it is tempting to join in and go along. In fact, if we are around negative energy it will rub off on us, and soon we will find ourselves sharing this negative attitude. But most of the time those negative ideas and conversations do not serve us. On the other hand, many people have an interesting experience when they really focus on staying positive. They often find that some friends are so negative that they have little to talk about with them anymore, and as time moves on and they maintain the positive vibration, they can actually attract more positive people in their lives! The positive-vibration people find they are spending more and more time around that energy, and in fact this supports their own positive energy! Gratitude awakens us to unlimited possibilities, and the belief in unlimited possibilities is the definition of hope, which can translate perfectly into perfect health. The more time we spend being grateful for the health we have, no matter if we have excellent health or poor health, the more positive we will feel and the more hope we will experience. A grateful attitude shows us that even if we can't see a perfectly straight and easy path to our goal of good health, we are grateful for whatever health we have. This is why so many former cancer patients, or those who have suffered tremendous health-related trials and illnesses, go on to become active in supporting others who are going through similar situations. They know what it is like, they have traveled the same road, and consequently they can give tremendous hope to the sick or injured person. These former patients know this, and while it might seem more logical that they would want to move on and put their experiences behind them, a large percentage of patients instead volunteer to support others who need their positive energy.

Changing our subconscious thoughts to ones of hope and gratitude can be achieved by anyone, at anytime, anywhere. It doesn't matter who we are, or what our incomes or situations are. If we let ourselves accept and believe these new thoughts in our conscious minds and hold them in our subconscious minds, they will guide us through our lives with very different results. Think of what this can do for our health. A person with a positive mind-set expects favorable thoughts and ideas, and they get them. As the stickperson diagram showed us in Chapter 1, we can consciously choose these positive thoughts. A positive conscious mind literally attracts happiness and joy. These emotions are deposited into the subconscious mind over time, and this makes it easier to remain in a positive vibration long term. So, for example, if we are fighting an illness and we maintain a positive attitude, our minds will anticipate only success. We can't perceive, nor will we accept, failure. We can only win because whatever the mind perceives, it receives.

Unfortunately, not everyone can maintain positive thoughts. Remember the story of Beth, the woman who looked at everything as bad news? She was the one who complained over the nurses turning on and off the lights and thought everything in her life was horrible? She was one of the many people discussed in this book who didn't believe in the power of positive thought, and she is not alone.

Many people think this subject is nonsense. They ask, "How can something as simple as positive thoughts change my health and my life?" It does seem too good to be true, but why? Why does something simple have to be too good to be true? It is simple, but not easy. It's not always easy to change our perceptions and be grateful. First we must accept responsibility for our thoughts, and then we must change our thoughts in the conscious mind, which then change our emotions in our subconscious mind. The body then enters a new, more energetic and healthy vibration. This leads to the attraction of positive things in our world, and this will all show up in our actions and the results we ultimately achieve in *all* aspects of our lives.

If positive thought has been proven effective, then why don't more people learn how to use it? Although there are many people who accept this thought process as the truth, and they understand that it does work and that it can vastly improve our health, not many individuals know how to effectively use it to get their best results. Our subconscious minds are programmed from a long time ago, and it takes a lot of energy to change that old conditioning and get rid of the limiting beliefs we hold as truth in our subconscious minds. Intellectual factors are the way we can change our thoughts, and the their development is really the secret. The majority of people rely on their senses to influence their conscious minds, but the people who develop their intellectual factors can and do create any life they choose.

In fact, how many people do we know who say, "Think positive," when someone around them is having a bad day? That type of flippant attitude is not what we're talking about, and frankly this is a very good way to invalidate someone's feelings. It's become a cliché, "Think positive," and, unfortunately, when something becomes a cliché it is no longer accepted as real and sincere.

A physician friend of mine told me of a situation where he was treating two women for strep infections. Their symptoms were actually identical, but their attitudes were grossly different. One woman came in terribly upset, shouting at the doctor and the nurses, telling them how much pain she was in, that she needed medicine. She told the doctor that this sort of thing always happened to her. "It was just my luck," she said. "My daughter went off and got married to some guy in Vegas behind my back, and didn't even mention it to me. They just went off and did it. Of course, my husband doesn't support my feelings at all. And then at work they are laying off people, and I was certain I would be next because it always happens that way. Although I didn't get laid off, I did get reassigned to a department where I have to work in the basement, filing forms all day. Can you imagine how terrible that is?"

The story continued like this. One negative thing after the other. She thought she was cursed and that bad luck followed her everywhere. (Do you know someone like this?) The doctor started her on medication, and it took a week for her to begin to feel better. I believe her vibration was in such a negative state the medication couldn't penetrate the source of the infection easily.

The other woman, on the other hand, came in and was pleasant. She smiled at the doctor and at the nurses. Her attitude was better and her vibration was markedly higher. Even the way she held herself was a bit different. Her hair was salt and pepper, but she kept it long, nearly halfway down her back, tied in a loose ponytail. The doctor asked her what she was doing prior to the infection, if she had gone anywhere different, changed her lifestyle or anything.

"No, not really," she said. "Just gardening and things like that when I get home from work."

My friend asked her if she lived with anyone.

"No, I live alone," she said. "I enjoy it. Sometimes I get a bit lonely, but I have beautiful garden and am grateful I get to enjoy it so much. When I get home from work, I can go out into my own garden and cut flowers and pick vegetables. This really relaxes me, and I totally enjoy my quiet time. I am hopeful you will give me some medication, and I will be right back in my garden again soon! So really, what's the big deal?"

The second woman left the hospital two days later, five days before the other. My friend and I were discussing the difference in the cases, and we both agreed it had to do with positive attitude and the power that comes with the vibration of our body. We can even see it in the work they do. The first woman focused only on negative thoughts, which put her body into a negative vibration that directly affected her ability to heal quickly. I believe her negative attitude and expectation also directly resulted in her daughter getting married without her (who would want all that negative energy at their wedding anyway!), her unresponsive husband, and her new job in the basement (no one wanted to be around her!). The second woman wasn't monetarily wealthy. She was single. She lived alone. All of these things could possibly drive a person into negativity, but she refused to let this negativity enter her conscious mind. Instead she focused on what she was grateful for and the joy she had in her life. She found happiness in her garden, picking flowers, and being outside. She was choosing different thoughts to hold in her conscious mind, therefore her results were very different. So it was no surprise to us that she was out of the hospital five days before the other woman.

The power we have in choosing our thoughts is immense. When we are in a positive vibration, we attract pleasant feelings and constructive images. The second woman from the story saw her life as simple and happy and she lived in great gratitude. She saw her life as bright. It had more energy and more happiness. This manifested itself in every aspect of her life in the realm of good will and success. The treating physician definitely saw the difference in her health, the way it affected her, and the way she was able to rebound so quickly. Gratitude and hope allowed her to recover quicker.

The following is another story that I have heard and demonstrates this point very well. I am honestly not certain if this is true, but the point of this story if absolutely priceless.

Two men, both seriously ill, occupied the same hospital room. One man was allowed to sit up in his bed for an hour each afternoon to help drain the fluid from his lungs. His bed was next to the room's only window. The other man had to spend all his time flat on his back. The men talked for hours on end. They spoke of their wives and families, their homes, their jobs, their involvement in the military service, and where they had been on vacation.

Every afternoon, when the man in the bed by the window could sit up, he would pass the time by describing to his roommate all the things he could see outside the window. The man in the other bed began to live for those one-hour periods where his world would be broadened and enlivened by all the activity and color of the world outside. The window overlooked a park with a lovely lake. Ducks and swans played on the water while children sailed their model boats. Young lovers walked arm in arm amid flowers of every color, and a fine view of the city skyline could be seen in the distance. As the man by the window described all this in exquisite details, the man on the other side of the room would close his eyes and imagine this picturesque scene.

One warm afternoon, the man by the window described a parade passing by. Although the other man could not hear the band, he could see it in his mind's eye as the gentleman by the window portrayed it with descriptive words. Days and weeks passed.

One morning, the day nurse arrived to bring water for their baths only to find the lifeless body of the man by the window, who had died peacefully in his sleep. She was saddened and called the hospital attendants to take the body away.

As soon as it seemed appropriate, the other man asked if he could be moved next to the window. The nurse was happy to make the switch, and after making sure he was comfortable, she left him alone. Slowly, painfully, he propped himself up on one elbow to take his first look at the real world outside. He strained to slowly turn to look out the window beside the bed, and to his amazement he saw only a brick wall.

The man asked the nurse what could have compelled his deceased roommate to describe such wonderful things outside this window. The nurse responded that the man was blind and could not even see the wall. She said, "Perhaps he just wanted to encourage you." He saw the beauty in his mind and shared it.

We can be that blind man whenever we choose. We can see a life filled with hopes and dreams, or we can see a blank wall.

Hope provides encouragement for our patients. The power of encouragement through any crisis is critical. Without encouragement the patient begins to lose hope very quickly. Think about when we are sick. We perceive that it will never end, and time seems to go slower than ever. Now remember when we were children and we got to stay home from school because we were sick and our moms or dads stayed with us and brought ice cream and soup and read to us. Being sick was almost fun. Now I'm not saying illness is a blessing, but with encouragement and support, illness is easier to overcome and more easily tolerated by the patient.

To accomplish everything we've talked about, we must train ourselves and practice this thinking. It doesn't just happen overnight. But as we practice and grow we will choose positive thoughts for our conscious minds so the positive new outlook will eventually take over our subconscious minds. And soon we won't even have to think about it. Our paradigm will be changed! Suddenly the air will smell fresher, the sky bluer, our health will be perfect. And it will stay that way.

To believe in ourselves and our ability to be healthy and stay healthy we must always visualize only favorable scenarios. We have to block the idea that we will get sick soon. We must believe that we are healthy people, and think about our good health repeatedly so it can begin to develop in our subconscious minds. We must focus on using positive words in our inner dialogue and when talking with others. I use a gratitude journal so every day the first thing I write is about all of the things I am grateful for. This causes me to focus on the good in every situation. I am an avid cross-fitness trainer. My workouts are intense, and I frequently have to use a lot of positive energy and visualization to complete them. Some days after I have a really intense workout when I am physically sore, I write in my journal that I am grateful for the sore arms or legs because the soreness reminds me that I *have* arms and legs, and I am grateful that they are getting stronger.

To smile is like seeing a rainbow sometimes. We need to remember to smile more and smile at everyone. We'll be shocked at how this affects people. Think about when we're walking down the street and a stranger looks at us with no expression. That void of emotion on their face is the same thing as a frown or a grimace. On the other hand, don't we feel incredible when some random person smiles at us, and not just some inauthentic smile, but a real, genuine smile? We want to talk to this person. We want to ask them their name. We are picking up their positive energy. Smiling makes all the difference.

That optimistic attitude will reflect itself to our health. If we are happy, a common cold doesn't seem like a big deal; in fact, to an optimistic, hopeful person, a cold might be a great excuse to snuggle up on the sofa and take in a good movie or sleep in a little later. The world and everything in it changes when we're happy. Be persistent with this and we will stay healthy and be happy.

We often see the saying, "Live, Laugh, Love," on plaques and paintings. Laughter releases chemicals within the body that make us feel good and even can help us heal. Making a point to laugh often—even about the small things—can assist in a patient's overall state of mind and positive attitude. This in turn allows them to heal faster and be more vibrant.

We can also experience tremendous happiness when we make others happy, despite our own situations. Shared grief is half the sorrow, but happiness when shared is doubled. If we want to feel rich, just count all the things we have that money can't buy. The power of gratitude can't be underestimated.

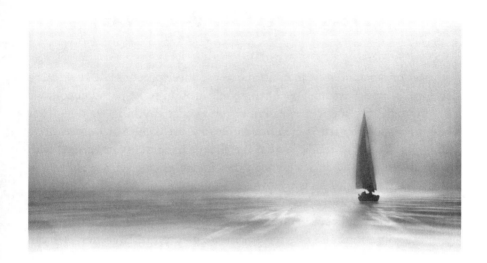

Chapter Twelve

—Your New, Healthier Life—

Within you right now is the power to do things you never dreamed possible. This power becomes available to you just as soon as you can change your beliefs.

—Dr. Maxwell Maltz

Chapter Twelve

To better understand how to continue to use these practices it is critical to develop a support system. We have people around to help and encourage us. Although this support is essential for almost anything we do in our lives, it is especially true when our bodies are weakened or our health is failing. But I want to reinforce that the change in thinking must start with us. We have to be the ones who want the change, encourage it, maintain it, and keep our thoughts focused toward our goals. As we have discussed, the first step is to allow only positive thoughts into our conscious minds. This will then directly affect our emotions and beliefs and it will ultimately show up in our vibrations and our results. As we gain more awareness, we can use the universal laws to help bring solutions and needed encouragement our way. But sometimes we need that extra little boost, and it can be hard to see the hope in a difficult situation.

Life coaching, or personal coaching, may be helpful as we are going through very difficult or traumatic times in our lives. A life coach can help us focus our thoughts and decide what dreams we really want to achieve. It can also provide accountability and bring us back to a positive vibration if we slide back into negative thought patterns.

I have functioned as a coach for many people on an informal basis due to my profession, and I have also had extensive training in personal and professional coaching, and I think that it's important to illustrate exactly what a life coach is. A life coach is someone to help us with and through our journey of personal development and growth. The coach helps us view things we are experiencing from an outside perspective and also helps us set goals for improvement in various areas. A coach helps us to reach our highest potential simply by helping us to change our perception and sometimes to gain clarity and focus.

As we change our thoughts and reach milestones that we have set, having a life coach is a great way to maintain our improvement and help encourage us to greater heights. When we attempt to accomplish a large goal on our own, it is very easy to fall back into our old thinking, which I call our comfort zone. A coach can help us get through our terror barrier!

During coaching we gain the skills and ideas that we can then use in the future long after the coaching period is complete. While there are intense short-term benefits that can create substantial change, we also learn the tools necessary to make continued long-term progress. When we hire a life coach we are investing in a higher level of us. Increased performance and life fulfillment are difficult goals, and there is a shorter learning curve if we have someone to help us through the steps and show us the way.

When it comes to selecting a life coach, it's important to ask around and then research various coaches. It is important to find someone who is compatible with our background and beliefs that can still open us to new ideas and methods of accomplishing what we want for our lives. We can choose a coach that we know and like, one that is well respected. But don't be fooled by thinking that the correct life coach needs to be someone who is just like us. Much of the time, the opposite is true. Sometimes the best coach is someone who is quite different from us but still someone we can trust. The most important factor is that they are willing and able and dedicated to us and our vision. The coach should have demonstrated success in his or her life. Just think about it—would we take investment advice from someone who had no money? They why would we hire a life coach who is unsuccessful and has a negative attitude? Look for the qualities in the coach that we value and are looking to achieve. A fitness coach should be in good physical shape, and a life coach should be in good mental shape!

It is important to start changing our thoughts even prior to beginning coaching so we can already have our positive mind-set in place. If we are not open to improvement, no amount of coaching will help. Remember the glasses we look through that color how we see our lives? What are you looking through? Do you see joy and hope, or do you see despair and hopelessness? All the same techniques of positive thought apply; if we feel that this endeavor is going to be rewarding, then it will be; if not, then it won't. We call this being coachable. We need to be in a positive vibration to attract positive thoughts to us, and our positive attitude will directly affect the coaching process. So if we feel that this coach will help us, then she will. As always, be grateful for the experience and you will be surprised as the good emerges from the coaching experience.

The main reason life coaching works is that our coach will have more experience than us in a certain areas of life improvement. He or she will also simply have a different perspective or point of view to look at our situations. For example, a little child doesn't ask their baby sibling for advice on how to throw a baseball; they watch and learn from someone who can do it. The same is the case with life coaching. Your coach can quickly identify patterns and signs that you might completely over look. Once these patterns and signs are identified, the coach will help you find the best solutions. Working well with a life coach can be one of the fastest ways to change your thinking and change your life.

The results experienced by most people who go through one-on-one coaching are incredible. A new person emerges and takes shape in a matter of weeks. We gain back that confidence that can sometimes wane when we have to deal with problems and suffer through setbacks alone. It is also helpful to seek coaching even when things are going well. Even as we have successes, it is still helpful to have encouragement and someone to help push us even higher. The intellectual factors are like muscles and need to be developed. Even the best athletes still train with a coach, so we should train our minds with a coach as well.

To give us an idea of how a typical coaching session works and how we can apply it to our health, here is an example:

During a period of time when a patient of mine, Kevin, was going through a relatively stressful time in his life, not only in his health but virtually every other area as well, he decided to consult a life coach. He had already gone through the process of forming a better, more positive mind-set.

Kevin believed that everything he wanted to accomplish would eventually happen. Once he was on this path he felt he might need a bit of help to maintain that sense of confidence. He also wanted to solve some bigger, overarching challenges in his life.

Kevin knew I was a LifeSuccess consultant and asked my opinion of how he could maintain this optimistic attitude despite having some pressing challenges. I suggested a life coach, and after a bit of research, Kevin found one that worked well for him. He really enjoyed the sessions and was happy with the coaching he received. He was able to see a different way to look at his situation. The coach shared some incredibly helpful and creative problem-solving skills, and he coached Kevin through various visualization drills where he could see the result before it happened, and how he could change his conscious thoughts and therefore change his paradigm, which in turn affected his results.

It is an important distinction that a life coach is not a therapist or counselor. Life coaches encourage their clients to find the answers that are the best for them by guiding the individual through the process of self discovery and by elevating their awareness level. Just as an athletic coach helps the athlete achieve his highest potential, so does a life coach, but with the latter he is working on achieving a higher level in all aspects of his life.

I asked Kevin, after some time had passed, how the coaching was going. "Great," he said. "We work mostly on my professional challenges, but also on the personal stuff, too." He later told me that his teaching was going smoother than ever. The homework was done and graded before he left for the day, the kids were more inquisitive, and his relationships with his friends and family were more fulfilling. The coach especially helped him deal with the importance of intuition in life. Since he had in fact used the intellectual factors as tools to help him achieve his dreams and goals, Kevin was happier and felt more in harmony with life. He found that he was able to hear his intuition for the first time.

When we change the way we think, our results will change.

Dr. Marianne Urbanski

Live Life to Its Fullest

When we accept that we control everything in our lives through our thoughts, feelings, and actions, we can't help but share this with others. This is one of the many ways we can live our lives to the fullest. I like to think of it as my gift to the world—to share a positive attitude with everyone I meet. The interesting thing is that since I have had this attitude, I attract and interact with more positive, happy, and grateful people. The vibration that we give off is exactly what returns to us.

We can touch other people's lives by simply allowing positive thoughts to come into our conscious minds, and sharing our positive vibrations with everyone we meet. We can leave people with joy and gratitude, thus giving them positive thoughts. We can also teach them what we've learned, even if it is something incredibly small, like smiling to a stranger on the bus, or saying good morning to someone we don't know. It is the smallest acts of kindness, I really believe, that are sometimes the most profound.

I was in New York City a few months ago, riding the subway. It was one of those terribly hot days, a day where the temperature had already reached 85 degrees by eight in the morning and not a cloud in the sky. It was one of those days that remind me of the song lyrics, "Hot time, summer in the city ..." The subway car windows didn't open and were dripping with wetness so much that we couldn't see outside anymore. It was a Monday, and so of course the people were angry and tired and clearly did not want to be riding a subway in the middle of Manhattan. I looked around and saw all of their faces. Not one smiling. They were all sending out negative vibrations.

I was sitting next to a woman in a suit and glanced at her only briefly. She was not smiling or talking, so I didn't press conversation. She didn't look angry, just appeared quiet. We both got off at the same stop and walked to the same coffee house. There was a gentleman working behind the counter and he was clearly having a bad day. He was rude and short answered, never smiling, even as I paid for my coffee. I smiled at the man, but it seemed to have no effect. The woman who sat next to me on the bus watched me, and then also smiled at the man and then thanked him for the coffee. She wished him a nice day. The guy behind the counter didn't say anything to her either, really, just grunted a bit and helped the next customer.

I stood there thinking, she gets it. She was in my life so briefly, but I will always remember her and how we each gave one another a positive boost by doing nothing more than buying coffee. It's interesting to observe that like-minded people we briefly encounter can really have an impact on us and on our day.

Our interactions with people greatly impact not only the people that we come in contact with, but the ones they come in contact with and the ones they contact. It is like a ripple in a pond. (Remember the laws! Many are at work here!) We can control everything that comes into our minds and then reflect that upon others. People respond well to joy and happiness because most of the time they want that for themselves. When someone believes they cannot control what other people do and say, and therefore they feel it is useless to try, I suggest the following: If we pass our positive energy on to only one person, their day will most likely be changed. We will have impacted whether a part of their day was pleasant or not. We can make that choice. And that's what wonderful about this. We don't need to have a lot of money, be the best looking person in the world, or have the most prestigious job—this technique spans all borders and generations, and it seeps into everyone's life that chooses to accept it as truth.

People sometimes ask, so have you found the secret of life? Yes, I say! I have! And the best part is that it's something literally everyone can learn. We know that money isn't the key to happiness, more stuff isn't the key; winning the lottery or recognition and the chance to live a life with incredible financial wealth and worry isn't either, although all of these sound tempting. Money comes and money goes, but the real key is listening to ourselves and to our intuition. From this space we will have abundance in *all* aspects of our lives! When we live every day in gratitude we will find happiness and joy in whatever our situation. When we take responsibility for our own thoughts, everything we want will find its way to us. Change our thoughts and our lives will change. Take everything one step at a time and gain knowledge through repetition. In a short time, it will become second nature. When we do these things in a relaxed state, we will notice changes in all aspects of our lives.

If we put our dream of better health in our conscious minds, and continue to nurture this thought, and plant it firmly in our heart, and if we believe that we become what we think about, now we know that we **can** become that vibrant healthy person we dream of being, one thought at a time!